·EASY KETO·
DINNERS

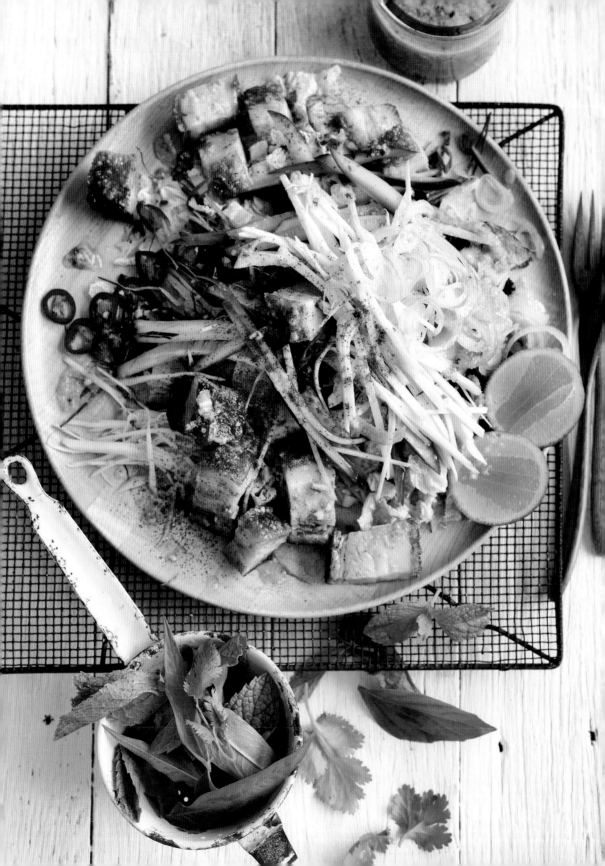

EASY KETO.

DINNERS

60+ SIMPLE KETO MEALS
FOR ANY NIGHT OF THE WEEK

PETE EVANS

plum. Pan Macmillan Australia

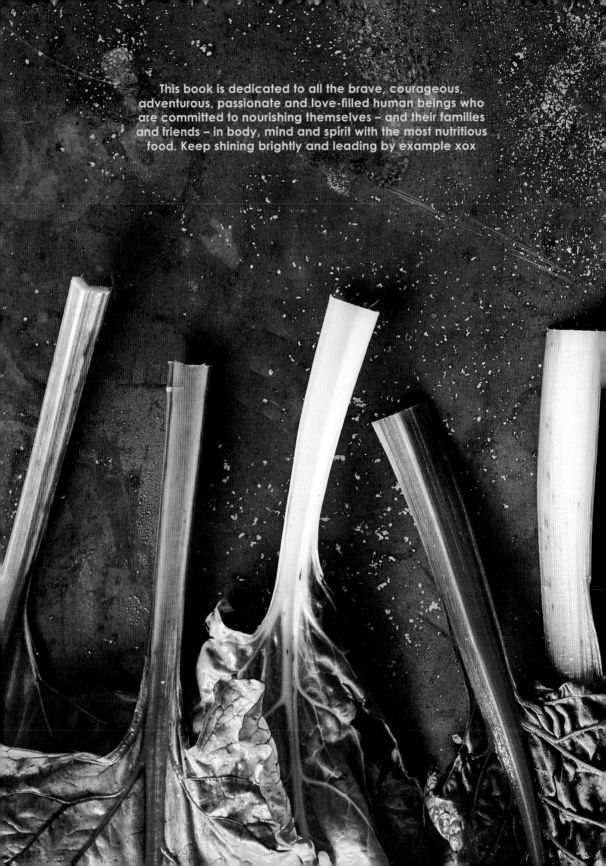

This book is dedicated to all the brave, courageous, adventurous, passionate and love-filled human beings who are committed to nourishing themselves – and their families and friends – in body, mind and spirit with the most nutritious food. Keep shining brightly and leading by example xox

CONTENTS

INTRODUCTION 6

GOING KETO 9

SEAFOOD 29

CHICKEN & DUCK 53

PORK 89

BEEF 111

LAMB 147

BASICS 163

GLOSSARY 180

THANKS 186

INDEX 188

INTRODUCTION

I cannot thank you enough for once again choosing the nourishing recipes and nutritional advice I love to share. Being Australia's top-selling cookbook author means so much to me, and at the same time illustrates that there is a genuine hunger to make the best choices we can to change our lives for the better. Sometimes helping and educating those you love most can feel like an uphill battle, but, believe me, trusting your actions and the way you live can only have a positive impact. After all, these lifestyle decisions have a ripple effect through to our families and friends, and then spread out to the wider community. Remember, if your main goal is to achieve good health and thrive, eating good-quality keto food will help you to lose weight, increase energy levels and improve cognitive function.

Which brings us to these wonderful keto dinners we have compiled for you and your loved ones. And when I say we, I mean all the members of my family, especially my wife Nic and my daughters Chilli and Indii – who try these dishes and add their input as we develop them – and the wonderful behind-the-scenes duo Monica and Jacinta Cannataci – who have worked with me for the last 13 years (since they were 19 years old!) in my restaurants and on every single cookbook we have produced over that time. All my creations are sent to Monica and Jacinta to execute and perfect. They test and retest the recipes so that every time you recreate one at home you can rely on it to be amazing.

Easy Keto Dinners is a flow-on from our *Easy Keto* handbook. Having listened to what you loved about the recipes in that collection, I wanted to inspire you further and make your time in the kitchen and around the table even more pleasurable. You asked for more simple dishes that would tempt even the fussiest of eaters without forgoing any flavour – and here they are! I know many of you face dietary challenges and that is why these recipes have a paleo theme as their foundation, excluding inflammatory grains and dairy and promoting a very healthy diet of animal fat/protein and vegetables. If you suffer from an autoimmune disease or have gut problems, you may wish to eliminate nuts, seeds, eggs and nightshades (tomatoes, potatoes, chillies, eggplants and capsicums), then reintroduce them one at a time to see how your body reacts.

Obviously, we encourage nutrient-dense whole foods and nose-to-tail eating from the very healthiest, naturally raised or caught land and sea animals. Think grass-fed and -finished herbivores (cattle, lamb, game); organic poultry (chicken and duck); free-range pigs; and wild-caught sustainable seafood (favouring smaller species like sardines, anchovies and mullet and farmed seafood like oysters, mussels, scallops, pipis and clams). When it comes to vegetables and fruit, we really need to choose organic where possible and avoid foods sprayed with the herbicide glyphosate (this barbaric practice is hurting not only ourselves but the planet at large). Never underestimate the power of the individual who is passionate about their choices; together we can bring about beneficial change.

Okay, now that we have that out of the way, in *Easy Keto* we outlined the essentials you need to go keto and included macronutrient percentages with the recipes. In *Easy Keto Dinners* I have decided not to include these, as I feel they can be too restrictive and may cause you to lose touch with what it actually means to enjoy your food. If, however, you want to track your macronutrients, then by all means go for it. I have never counted a carb, nor do I want to. I eat intuitively and that means I listen to my body – some days I eat one meal and on others I eat three; sometimes I snack and some days I fast for 24 hours or more. Each and every time I do this, I tune in to my body and what it wants. If that sounds strange, try out some of the ketogenic approaches I have listed (see page 10) for a week or more, then change it up and see how you feel. I love flexibility and I eat what I want and when I feel like it. So, for instance, I would say 90 per cent of the time I am in a state of ketosis (see page 9) and the other 10 per cent I break out of it while still sticking to paleo principles. For more information on those times when you are cycling out of ketosis and feel like a high-carb day, see page 12. My intention is maximum nourishment for my body, mind and spirit. But we are all different and I encourage you to experiment with when and what you eat to help you find the approach that works best for you.

All the delicious recipes in this book have been created to help you do just this. And even though I say they are dinners, sometimes my dinner is at midday (my last meal of the day) and sometimes dinner is my breakfast (my first and only meal of the day); these meals really are designed to be enjoyed at any time of day. I think it's time we forge a truly healthy relationship with food and break away from the notion of what breakfast, lunch or dinner should be and instead adopt a more intuitive approach. Your body will thank you for it!

Once again, thank you for your support and for helping to pave the way for a healthier future for the coming generations and the planet as a whole.

I love you all. Keep cooking and living with love and laughter.

Pete xo

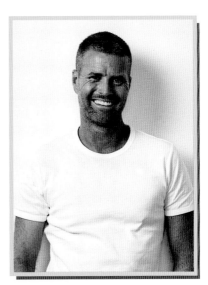

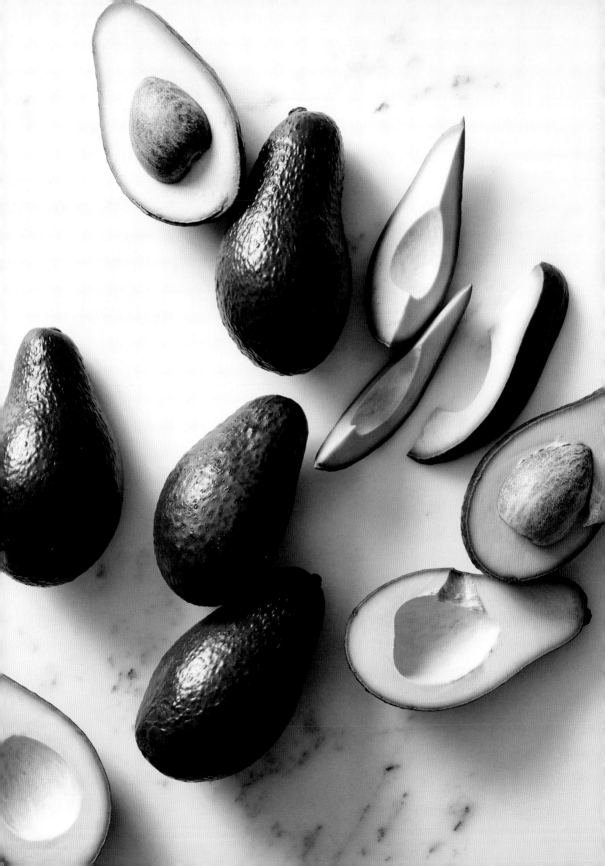

GOING KETO

A ketogenic diet is one that is low in carbs, relatively high in healthy fats and with moderate amounts of protein. It is sometimes combined with regular fasting. Eating this way forces the body to burn fat rather than glucose as its main source of energy, thereby entering a state known as ketosis.

Let me explain. The body's two main sources of energy are glucose and fat. When we eat a high-carb diet, our body converts the carbohydrates into glucose and uses that to provide the fuel we need to function. In order to switch our body from burning glucose to burning fat (ketosis), we need to significantly reduce the amount of carbohydrates we consume. When our body is in ketosis, the liver converts fatty acids into molecules called ketone bodies, which then travel to the brain where they are used as the main source of energy.

WHY CHOOSE KETO?

The ketogenic diet can have a whole range of benefits, including burning body fat and helping to lose weight, improving mental clarity and providing sustained energy. It is a tool that can be used throughout your life to support better overall health.

Going keto may also help to manage metabolism. When we eat healthy fats and sufficient good-quality protein, plus minimise our daily carb intake, it can help to significantly reduce hunger. This is because, no matter what build or weight we are, fat is abundant in our bodies, so once we switch over to burning fat for energy, there is a steady supply of fuel as long as we maintain a healthy diet. Fats and protein also have a positive effect on appetite-controlling hormones.

Furthermore, there is some evidence that the keto diet may assist with the prevention and management of metabolic disorders, including inflammatory disorders, such as polycystic ovarian syndrome and obesity, type 2 diabetes and cardiovascular disease.

The benefits of choosing keto:

- Balanced hormonal health.
- Improved mental clarity and focus.
- Improved metabolism.
- Long-lasting energy.
- Reduced appetite and decreased cravings.
- Reduced risk of chronic diseases.

CHOOSING YOUR KETOGENIC APPROACH

It is all about experimenting and finding what works best for you, as well as being flexible to allow for changes in your body due to ageing, health or level of exercise. Try keeping a food diary to write down what you eat at every meal and how you feel afterwards. If you like, you can follow up with blood and hormone tests with your healthcare professional. There are five main ketogenic approaches:

1. Full ketogenic
Adopt a very low-carbohydrate lifestyle (20–50 grams of net carbs per day), so you are in a constant state of ketosis.

2. Cyclical ketogenic
Cycle in and out of ketosis.
Consume a higher level of carbohydrates (50–150 grams per day) 1–2 days per week, fortnight or month.
Consume less than 50 grams of net carbs on the other days.
Mimics the hunter–gatherer feast/famine cycle.

3. Intuitive ketogenic
Stay in a state of ketosis most of the time.
Fluctuate in and out of ketosis.
No need to count carbs but always stick to low-carb foods.
Tune in to your body and respond to how you feel.

4. Targeted ketogenic
Eat all your carbs either before or after training.
Geared towards athletes and fitness enthusiasts.

5. Carnivore ketogenic
Reduce carbs altogether, increase protein intake to 35–45 per cent and reduce fat intake to 55–65 per cent.
May help to reduce hunger and inflammation.
Possible first step before transitioning to another approach.
Any of the recipes in this book can be adapted for this strategy by simply leaving out the vegetables and fruit.

I personally favour the intuitive ketogenic approach of staying in a state of mild ketosis and then fluctuating in and out as my body sees fit. I don't count carbs, but generally eat very low carb to lower carb with the occasional higher intake of carbs when I feel like it, without being regimented or following a strict program.

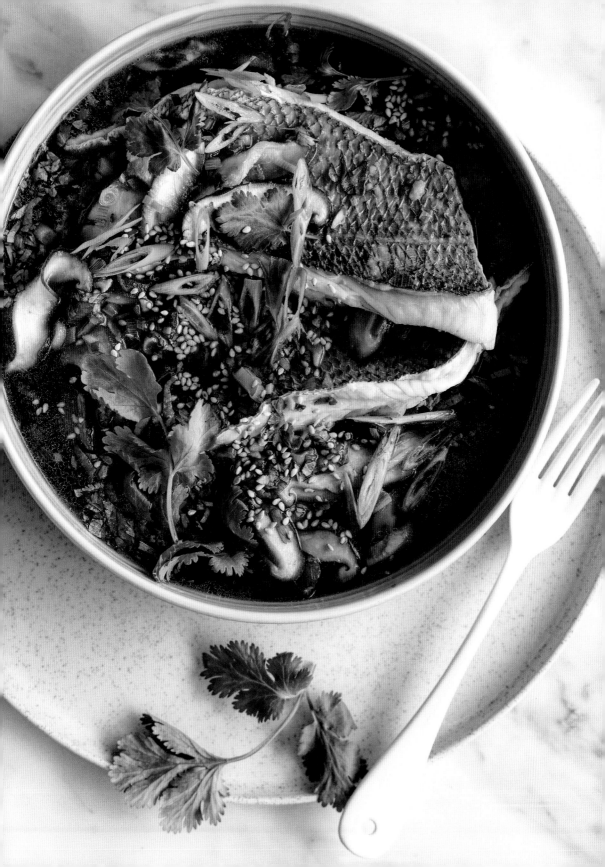

A GUIDE TO CYCLING IN AND OUT OF KETOSIS

A typical cyclical ketogenic diet is a matter of eating, feasting and fasting. By that I mean eating the right foods to put your body into ketosis; occasionally feasting (and cycling out of ketosis) by having a relatively high-carb day; and fasting intermittently.

EATING: HOW TO GO INTO KETOSIS

In order to enter a state of ketosis, you need to significantly reduce the amount of carbohydrates you eat so your body switches to burning fat, rather than glucose, for fuel. This is achieved by limiting your net carb intake to less than 50 grams per day (some people like to keep it closer to 20 grams per day).

Personally, I'm not one to count carbs, but it is something you may need to do until you understand the quantities required and the process becomes more intuitive. The majority of recipes in this book – with the exception of those with a 'HIGH-CARB DAY' symbol – are very low carb, and ideal for entering and maintaining a state of ketosis. You can also refer to the table on pages 20–21 showing the level of carbohydrates in common foods. Remember that most of your carbs should come from from non-starchy veggies and you should generally eat them with fat and protein.

Once you are consuming less than 50 grams of net carbs per day by eating this way, it can take anywhere from seven to 30 days for your body to enter ketosis (see page 17 for tips on how to know if you are in ketosis). Don't panic if it takes some time to happen – everybody is different. If you feel any 'keto slump' symptoms during this early transition period, see page 16 for tips on how to support your body through this time.

FEASTING: HOW TO CYCLE OUT OF KETOSIS

With a cyclical ketogenic approach, you will have a high-carb day (up to 150 grams of net carbs) every week, fortnight, month or season depending on what feels best for you. It's simply a matter of experimenting with the timing and frequency of your high-carb days, listening to your body. I usually fluctuate between 20 and 50 grams on most days, and then occasionally increase my carbs to 100–150 grams when I feel I need to.

Now, a high-carb day doesn't mean shovelling down potato chips, pizza, pasta, biscuits and other starchy foods that will simply convert to glucose and spike blood-sugar levels. You should still be avoiding foods that are most likely to cause inflammation, such as dairy, grains, legumes and refined sugars. Instead, enjoy some healthy carbohydrate-rich options, such as sweet potato, pumpkin, parsnip, carrot, beetroot or keto bread. Keep an eye out for the 'HIGH-CARB DAY' symbol on recipes in this book to use as a guide.

FASTING: A NATURAL COMPANION TO KETO

Once your body switches from carb-burning to fat-burning mode, you can usually go for longer periods without feeling hungry. For this reason, fasting tends to be a natural part of the ketogenic diet. If you do decide to fast, I recommend easing into it. Start with intermittent fasting, which limits your eating time to a 6–8-hour period. For example, if you have your first meal of the day at 10 am, your last meal will be before 6 pm. This means you are fasting for 16–18 hours between meals. For women, some nutritionists recommend fasting for 14–15 hours or less, though there are also many women who thrive on 16–18 hours.

If possible, start by setting aside one day a week to fast intermittently. Eat your last meal before 6 pm in the evening and don't have your next meal until 10 am or 12 pm on the following day. Once you get used to this, you can try intermittent fasting seven days a week. Depending on what I am doing, I often eat only one or two meals a day. Generally, my first meal of the day is around 2–4 pm, with perhaps a broth in the morning. Sometimes I go 48 hours without eating and instead drink water and bone broth. At other times, such as when I am on a surfing holiday, I am more than happy to eat three meals a day to meet my body's demands. The key is always to be flexible, listen to your body and adapt the food you eat accordingly.

It's important to note that fasting is not the right option for everyone. Make sure you discuss it with your healthcare professional before you start, especially if you have type 2 diabetes, hormonal imbalances, kidney disease or cancer. Fasting is not recommended for babies, children, teenagers, the elderly or pregnant or breastfeeding women.

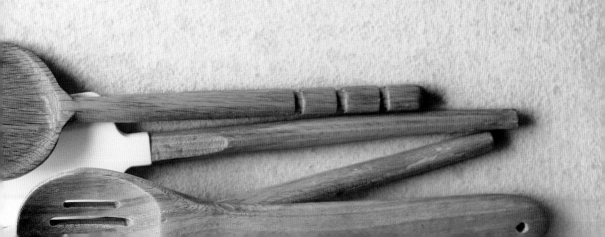

GETTING STARTED

1. REMOVE REFINED CARBS
Spend a few days, weeks or even months eliminating refined sugar, grains and grain-based foods, such as pasta and bread, from your diet before you transition to keto. Once your carbs are coming from healthy sources, such as vegetables, nuts and seeds, you can play around with different levels of carbs, fat and protein to see what works best for your body.

2. EMBRACE HEALTHY FATS
Keto is all about replacing carbohydrates with good-quality healthy oils and fats. For cooking, I use coconut oil – which can withstand high temperatures – as well as lard, tallow, ghee and chicken and duck fat. For salad dressings and drizzling over finished dishes, I recommend olive, macadamia and avocado oils.

Organic grass-fed meat, pastured eggs, wild-caught seafood, avocados, nuts and seeds are also excellent sources of healthy fats. Raw cacao butter is great too – I use it in baking and smoothies. I also love MCT (medium-chain triglycerides) oil, which contains a special type of saturated fatty acid that is easily digested to provide fast, sustained energy. I add it to smoothies and salad dressings. For more information on which fats to include when going keto, see pages 24–25.

3. EAT ENOUGH PROTEIN
As well as helping us to feel full for longer, protein is an essential building block for the body and plays an important role in helping to regulate its processes. I recommend getting roughly 25 per cent of your daily energy from protein (with 70 per cent from fat and 5 per cent from carbs). However, as always, this can differ from person to person, so it's important to pay attention and keep flexible. I always choose the fattiest cuts of meat and seafood, as they are cheaper and more flavoursome, and are also a great way of boosting your fat intake to help your body go into ketosis.

4. KEEP HYDRATED
This is very important, as water is a natural appetite suppressant and hydration helps to promote weight loss. Headaches, muscle cramps and weakness occur if there is inadequate hydration. Adjusting your salt intake can help with electrolyte imbalance – I recommend drinking a cup of bone broth a day (or every few days) and including good-quality unrefined sea salt or Himalayan salt in your diet.

5. BOOST KEY MINERALS
Key minerals, such as iodine and magnesium, are very important when transitioning to a keto diet, as they help to boost energy and also play a supportive role in the hormonal, digestive and neurological systems. Include sea vegetables, such as seaweed, in your diet to make sure you are getting enough iodine. Avocado, nuts and seeds and oily fish all contain magnesium, but adding magnesium flakes to the bath is the most efficient means of boosting your intake as it is best absorbed through the skin.

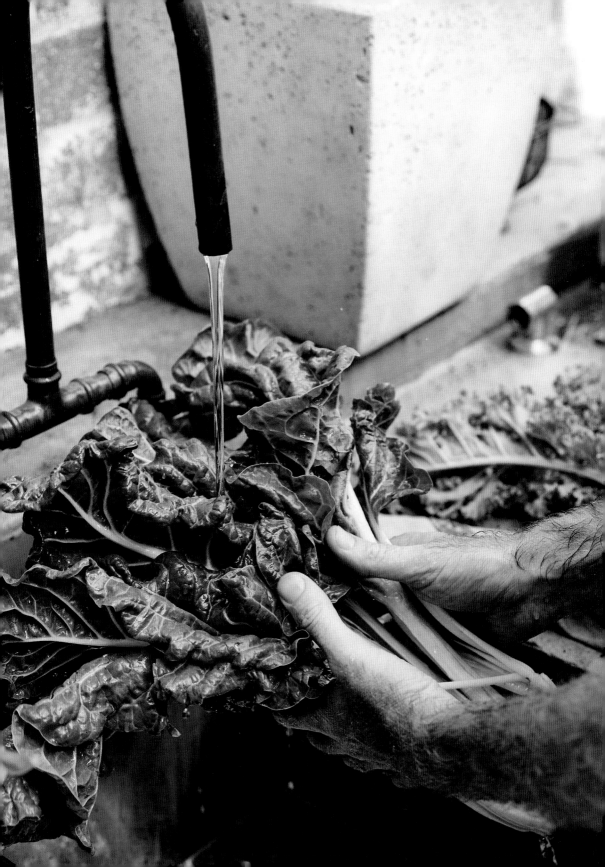

HOW TO AVOID THE KETO SLUMP

Adopting a keto diet involves a big shift in how the body functions – from short, sharp sugar burning to slow, sustained fat burning – and can take a bit of getting used to. The first 3–4 weeks (and sometimes longer, depending on your state of health) are always the hardest. During this time, you may experience what is known as 'keto flu', with symptoms including headaches, brain fog, exhaustion, constipation, diarrhoea, dizziness and irritability. To help prevent this from happening, here are some easy steps to take:

GET PLENTY OF HYDRATION
Drink the purest filtered water possible – around 2 litres a day is good, but listen to your body.

UP THE ELECTROLYTES
You may wish to increase your salt intake to 2 teaspoons of unrefined sea or Himalayan salt, and include 300–400 milligrams of magnesium and 1–2 grams of potassium each day for a period of time. Going keto really flushes out water weight and, as a result, electrolytes.

ENJOY DAILY (GENTLE) EXERCISE
Whether it's walking, swimming, cycling, dancing, practising yoga or just walking the dog, low-level, gentle exercise is the perfect companion to going keto.

EAT LOW-CARB VEGGIES AND FRUIT
Raspberries, blackberries, strawberries and blueberries are all relatively low in sugar and chock full of phytonutrients. Make sure they are organic and spray free.

GET ADEQUATE REST AND SLEEP
Try mind-calming techniques, such as breathing and meditation, and avoid spending too much time in front of electronic devices before bed.

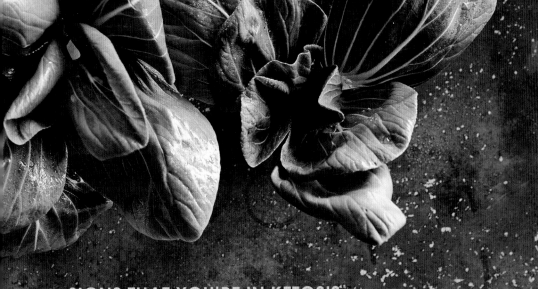

SIGNS THAT YOU'RE IN KETOSIS

Here are the key signs to look out for:

IMPROVED MENTAL CLARITY AND FOCUS

The dramatic swings you notice in energy and performance when eating a diet high in carbs do not happen when you are in a state of ketosis. Some people even experience a feeling of euphoria once in ketosis.

CONTROLLED HUNGER AND NO MORE CRAVINGS

Your body has a constant ready supply of energy when burning fat rather than glucose for fuel. The healthy fats in your diet also help you feel satiated for longer.

SUSTAINED ENERGY

It takes roughly 90 minutes for your body to use up the energy from eating carbs before starting to 'crash'. This doesn't happen when you're in a state of ketosis because your body is running off an almost limitless source of fuel.

INCREASED THIRST AND A METALLIC TASTE IN THE MOUTH

Your body uses up excess glycogen and increases urination when transitioning to a keto diet, which means you'll probably be pretty thirsty unless you up the electrolytes (see opposite). You may also experience a metallic taste in your mouth.

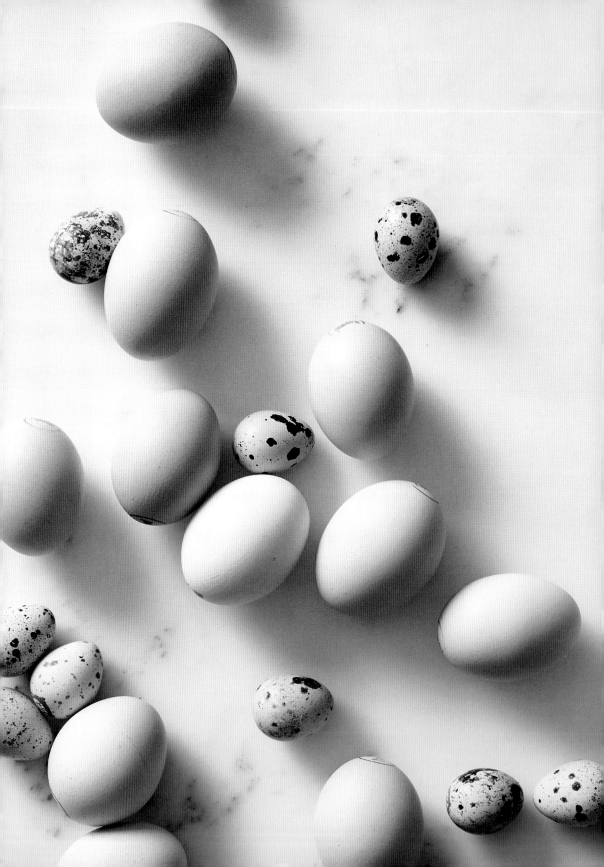

CARBS FOUND IN COMMON FOODS AND DRINKS

It can be helpful to measure your net carbohydrate intake when first transitioning to a ketogenic diet. The table on pages 20–21 shows the net carbs found in the foods and drinks most commonly consumed when following a keto diet.

THE DIFFERENCE BETWEEN NET CARBS AND TOTAL CARBS

When going keto, a common mistake is to count the *total* carbs in foods instead of the *net* carbs, leading to a restriction of foods high in dietary fibre. Instead, we should subtract the fibre from the total carb count, because fibre is an indigestible carbohydrate that isn't absorbed into our system and therefore doesn't affect our blood sugar. To work out the net carbs, just subtract the fibre from the total carbs. For example, 100 grams of almonds contains 22 grams of total carbs and 12 grams of fibre, so the net carb count is 10 grams.

TOTAL CARB COUNT – FIBRE COUNT = NET CARBS

MACRONUTRIENTS AND COUNTING CARBS

Because people's bodies are so different in the way they metabolise food, I think it's important to not get too prescriptive over the exact macronutrient percentages in meals. It is generally more useful to look at your approximate macro breakdown for the whole day rather than obsessing over the macros of each individual meal.

The same goes for counting carbs. While you may need to count carbs when you first start out, to make sure you are consuming the 20 to 50 grams of net carbs to be in ketosis, it's not helpful to get stressed about whether you've had 35 or 35.5 grams of carbohydrates that day. The figures in the table overleaf are estimations only – the exact amount of carbohydrates in ingredients can vary depending on where they are grown, whether they are in season and how you cook them.

Above all else, try to relax and listen to your body. Try a more intuitive approach by keeping a journal about what you eat and how you feel. Once you have been on a ketogenic diet for a while you will begin to understand when your body is in ketosis. You'll have more energy, feel clear-headed and you won't get hungry between meals. This is the best way to figure out if you're consuming the right carb, fat and protein ratios for your body. And remember, as long as you're cooking with nutrient-dense whole foods, including healthy fats and good-quality protein, and avoiding grains, legumes and dairy, you can't go too far wrong!

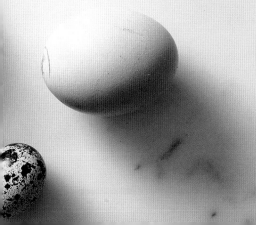

FOOD/DRINK	NET CARBOHYDRATES
Almonds (28 g)	3
Apple (100 g)	11
Artichokes (100 g)	1
Banana (100 g)	20
Blackberries (100 g)	5
Blueberries (100 g)	12
Bok choy (100 g)	1
Brazil nuts (28 g)	1
Broccoli (100 g)	4
Brussels sprouts (100 g)	5
Cabbage (100 g)	4
Capsicum (100 g)	4
Carrots (100 g)	7
Cashew nuts (28 g)	8
Cauliflower (100 g)	3
Celery (100 g)	2
Chia seeds (28 g)	2
Clams (100 g)	4
Coconut flour (28 g)	6
Coconut water (250 ml)	7
Cucumber (100 g)	3
Dates (100 g)	71
Egg (1 large)	<1
Fennel (100 g)	4
Fish (100 g)	0
Flaxseeds (28 g)	1
Kale (100 g)	6
Kombucha (250 ml)	7

FOOD/DRINK	NET CARBOHYDRATES
Liver (chicken) (100 g)	1
Macadamia nuts (28 g)	2
Meat (chicken, beef, pork) (100 g)	0
Mussels (100 g)	7
Okra (100 g)	4
Olives (28 g)	1
Onion (100 g)	8
Orange (100 g)	9
Oysters (100 g)	5
Parsnip (100 g)	13
Pecan nuts (28 g)	1
Pistachio nuts (28 g)	4
Pumpkin (100 g)	6
Pumpkin seeds (28 g)	3
Radish (100 g)	2
Raspberries (100 g)	6
Rocket (100 g)	2
Sesame seeds (28 g)	0
Silverbeet (100 g)	3
Spinach, raw (100 g)	1
Strawberries (100 g)	5
Sunflower seeds (28 g)	4
Sweet potato (100 g)	17
Tomatoes (100 g)	3
Unsweetened cacao powder (28 g)	6
Walnuts (28 g)	1
Zucchini (100 g)	2

THE KETO KITCHEN

PANTRY

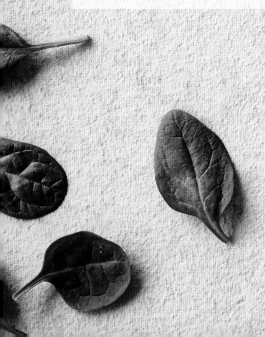

- Apple cider vinegar (raw)
- Cacao butter
- Cacao powder (raw and unsweetened)
- Coconut flour
- Coconut milk/cream
- Coconut, shredded
- Collagen powder (grass fed and marine)
- Dried herbs
- Fire tonic (medicinally spiced apple cider vinegar drink)
- Fish, jarred* (such as preserved anchovies, salmon, tuna, mackerel and sardines)
- Fish sauce
- Gelatine powder* (grass fed)
- Lemons and limes
- Nut and seed flours (such as almond meal)
- Nuts (almonds, macadamias, pecans, walnuts)
- Oils (coconut, extra-virgin olive, avocado, MCT)
- Salt* (unrefined varieties, such as sea, Himalayan)
- Seaweed (dulse, nori* and others)
- Seed crackers
- Seeds (chia, pumpkin, sunflower, sesame)
- Spices (turmeric, black pepper, paprika, cumin)
- Sprout seeds (broccoli, radish)
- Supplements (iodine, magnesium)
- Sweeteners* (liquid stevia, monk fruit, xylitol, erythritol, honey)
- Tahini
- Tamari/coconut aminos*
- Tomatoes, jarred (see Note page 66)
- Vanilla (pods, powder or paste)

FRIDGE

- Bacon, ham and salami (free range and nitrate free)
- Coconut yoghurt
- Curry pastes
- Dressings (homemade)
- Eggs (organic and free range)
- Fermented drinks (kombucha, dairy-free kefir)
- Fermented vegetables (kimchi, sauerkraut)
- Fish and shellfish
- Ghee (if choosing to include dairy)
- Good-quality animal fat* (lard, tallow, duck fat)
- Herbs (basil, parsley, mint, coriander)
- Kelp noodles and other sea vegetables
- Keto bread
- Low-carb fruits (blueberries, raspberries, blackberries, strawberries)
- Low-carb vegetables (cucumbers, celery, lettuce, tomatoes, silverbeet, cabbage, spring onions, radishes, cauliflower, broccoli)
- Mayonnaise
- Meats (all varieties, fattier cuts)
- Nut and seed butters
- Nut cheeses
- Nut milks (coconut, cashew and almond) and hemp milk
- Offal
- Olives
- Pâté
- Pickles
- Salmon roe/caviar
- Sprouts
- Sriracha chilli sauce
- Tomato ketchup

FREEZER

- Avocados (diced, for adding to smoothies and treats)
- Bananas (chopped, for adding to smoothies on high-carb days)
- Berries (blueberries, raspberries, blackberries, strawberries)
- Bone broth (beef, chicken, fish) (pages 165, 166 and 174)
- Bones for making broth
- Keto bread, sliced
- Leftovers (to ensure you always have something healthy to hand when you need to eat)
- Lemon and lime juice (frozen in ice-cube trays)

*See Glossary for more information on these ingredients

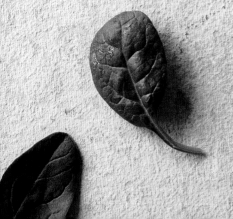

GOOD FATS ARE YOUR FRIENDS!

Fats provide us with energy and keep us feeling full for longer, as well as supplying us with vitamins A, D, E and K, and supporting the health of our nervous, immune and digestive systems. Animal fats and coconut oil are great for cooking, as they have high smoke points, while extra-virgin olive oil is wonderful in dressings and drizzled over dishes. If you choose to use dairy-based fats, ghee is the best option as it has a high smoke point and the milk sugars and proteins are removed in the clarification process. Here are some of my favourite fats to use in the kitchen:

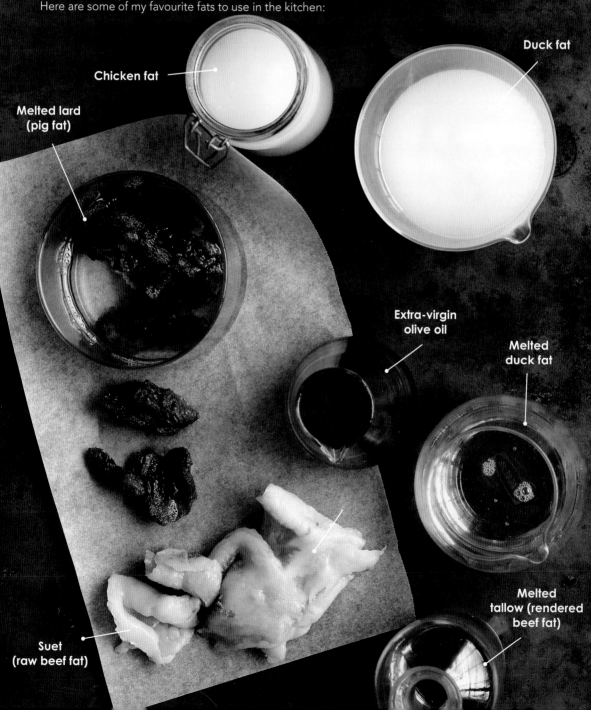

Chicken fat

Duck fat

Melted lard
(pig fat)

Extra-virgin
olive oil

Melted
duck fat

Melted
tallow (rendered
beef fat)

Suet
(raw beef fat)

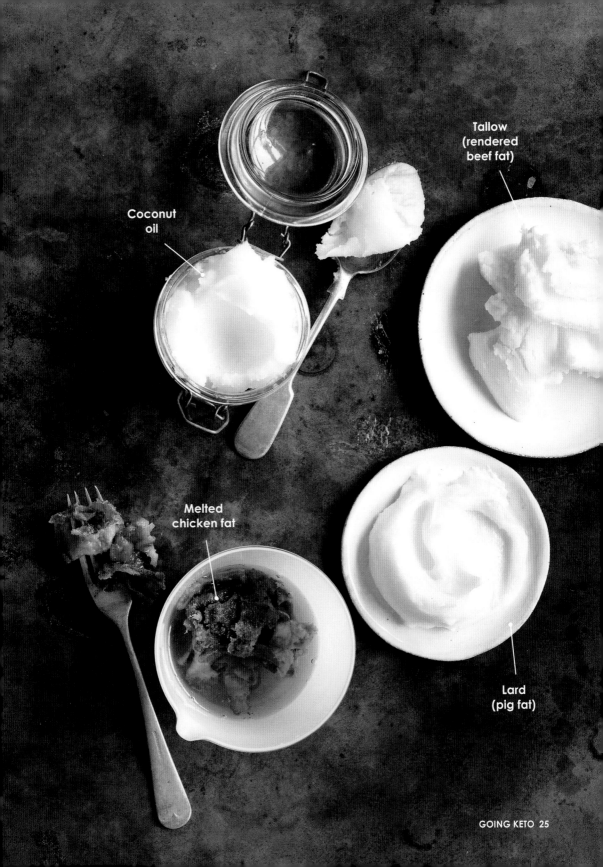

Coconut
oil

Tallow
(rendered
beef fat)

Melted
chicken fat

Lard
(pig fat)

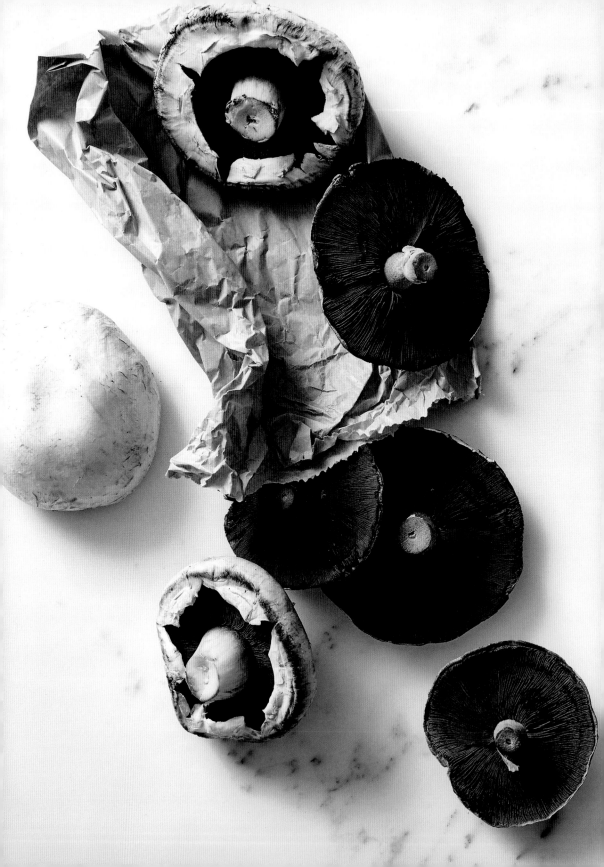

COMMON MEALS MADE KETO

Going keto starts with knowing where your food comes from and what's in it, so always read the labels and try to choose the most natural ingredients possible. Nurturing your health then becomes a matter of simple meal or ingredient swaps. Here are some ideas to get you started.

- **Burgers:** Replace grain-based rolls and burger buns with large field or portobello mushrooms, lettuce or cabbage leaves.

- **Cheese and crackers:** Replace wheat-based crackers and dairy-based cheese with flaxseed and chia seed crackers and nut or pumpkin cheese.

- **Hot chips:** Replace potato with zucchini or parsnip.

- **Pasta and noodles:** Replace grain-based pasta and noodles with spiralised vegetables (try zucchini, carrot and pumpkin) or kelp noodles.

- **Pizza:** Replace wheat-flour pizza bases with cauliflower pizza bases.

- **Sushi:** Replace white or brown rice with cauliflower or broccoli rice.

- **Tacos and tortillas:** Replace tacos and tortillas with lettuce, kale, cabbage or silverbeet leaves, or use cauliflower wraps.

- **Toasted sandwiches:** Replace grain-based breads with keto bread using almond meal or coconut flour instead of wheat flour.

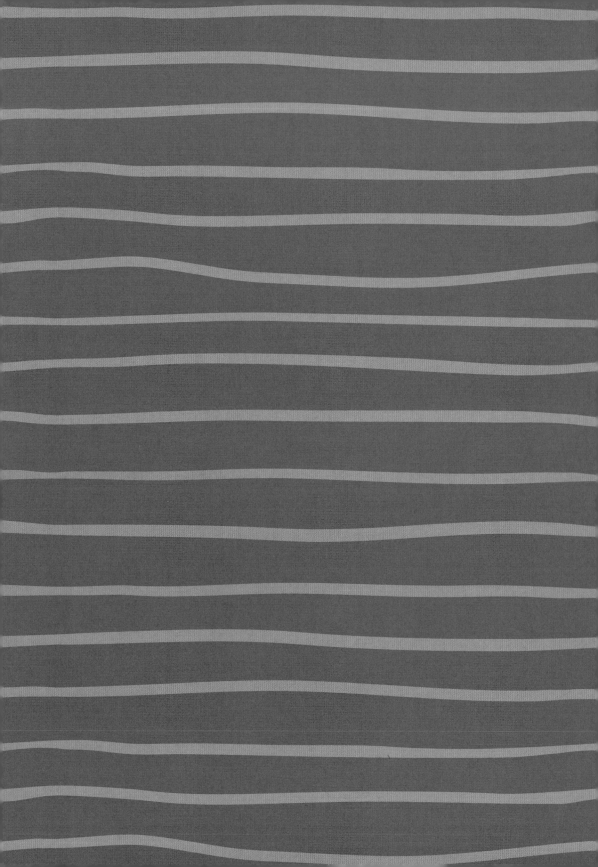

SEAFOOD

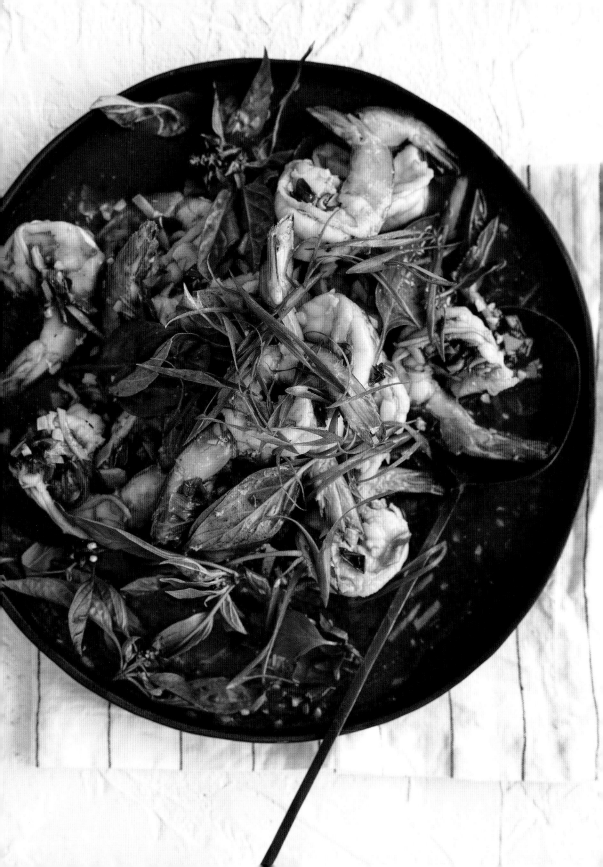

Ginger is one of the world's most-loved ingredients. It is definitely special to me and when I want a little bit of medicinal spice, I like to use it in many different ways, from drinks like homemade kombucha and kefir to treats and desserts. It is also great in any number of savoury dishes and works well with chicken, pork and seafood – especially prawns. With a minimum of fuss, this simple stir-fry will please everyone.

GINGER PRAWNS

Serves 2–4

3 tablespoons coconut oil or good-quality animal fat*
600 g raw prawns, shelled and deveined, tails left intact
5 cm piece of ginger, cut into fine matchsticks
4 spring onions, white parts chopped, green parts finely shredded
4 garlic cloves, finely chopped
2 bird's eye chillies, finely sliced
80 g gluten-free oyster sauce
1 tablespoon fish sauce
2 teaspoons coconut sugar
250 ml (1 cup) Brown Chicken Bone Broth (page 166)
sea salt and freshly ground black pepper
1 handful of Thai basil leaves

* See Glossary

Heat 1 tablespoon of the coconut oil or animal fat in a wok or large frying pan over medium–high heat. Add the prawns in batches and cook for 15 seconds on each side. Remove from the pan and set aside.

Wipe the pan clean, add the remaining oil or fat and place over medium–high heat. Add the ginger, spring onion whites, garlic and chilli and stir-fry for 2 minutes, or until fragrant and starting to colour slightly.

Combine the oyster sauce, fish sauce, coconut sugar and broth in a bowl, then pour into the pan and stir. Simmer for 1–2 minutes, or until the sauce thickens.

Return the prawns to the pan, add the spring onion greens and toss for about 30 seconds until the prawns are just cooked. Remove from the heat, season with salt and pepper, toss through the Thai basil leaves and serve.

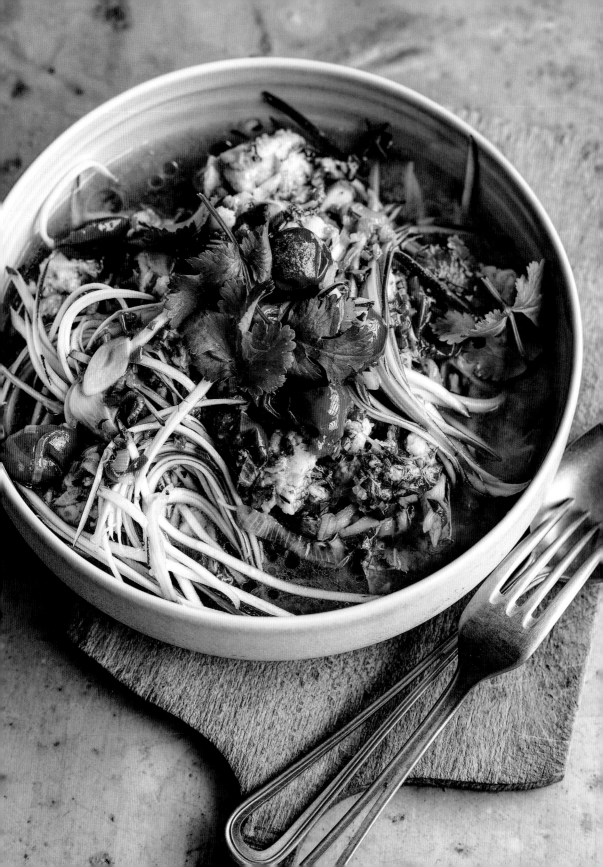

This is one dish I must have cooked tens of thousands of times when I owned my restaurant. In the restaurant, I used butter and fresh pasta, but these days I use paleo or keto noodles or spiralised vegetables instead. I have also changed the fat, but the end result is still amazing. If you can't find good-quality crabmeat, use fish or any other seafood you fancy.

BLUE SWIMMER CRAB LINGUINE

Serves 4

80 ml (⅓ cup) melted ghee or good-quality animal fat*
6 garlic cloves, sliced
4 French shallots, sliced
2 bird's eye chillies, finely chopped
1 bunch of coriander, roots, stalks and leaves chopped separately, plus extra sprigs to serve
3 tablespoons fish sauce
500 ml (2 cups) Brown Chicken Bone Broth (page 166)
24 cherry tomatoes, halved
4 large zucchini (about 600 g), spiralised into thin noodles
250 g cooked blue swimmer crabmeat
lime wedges, to serve

* See Glossary

Heat the ghee or fat in a large frying pan over medium heat. Add the garlic, shallot, chilli and chopped coriander root and sauté for about 5 minutes until just softened.

Add the fish sauce to the pan and cook for about 30 seconds to release the flavour. Tip in the broth and tomato halves, then increase the heat to medium–high and cook for 8–10 minutes until the sauce is reduced and thickened.

Add the zucchini noodles to the pan and toss through the sauce. Cook for 1 minute, then add the crabmeat and the rest of the chopped coriander. Serve with the coriander sprigs and a squeeze of lime.

Peas and trout are a marriage made in heaven. We make this at home from time to time as it brings a lot of joy to the dinner table. I love this dish for its good fats from the trout, its flavour and health-giving properties from the nourishing lemon broth, and the wonderful way the minted peas tie everything together. You could, of course, use salmon instead of trout, and feel free to add a poached egg if you want something even richer.

OCEAN TROUT WITH MINTED PEA PUREE AND LEMON BROTH

Serves 4

4 x 160 g ocean trout fillets, skin on, pin-boned
2 tablespoons coconut oil or good-quality animal fat*
1 tablespoon chopped mint leaves, plus extra leaves to serve

Lemon broth

1 tablespoon coconut oil or good-quality animal fat*
100 g speck, finely chopped
2 French shallots, chopped
500 ml (2 cups) Brown Chicken Bone Broth (page 166)
1 teaspoon finely grated lemon zest
3 teaspoons lemon juice
sea salt and freshly ground black pepper

Minted pea puree

350 g frozen peas, thawed
1 large handful of mint leaves
3 roasted or confit garlic cloves
3 tablespoons olive oil

* See Glossary

Preheat the oven to 200°C (180°C fan-forced).

To make the lemon broth, heat the coconut oil or animal fat in a saucepan over medium heat. Add the speck and shallot and cook for 5 minutes, or until lightly golden and softened. Pour in the broth, then stir though the lemon zest. Bring to the boil, reduce the heat to low and gently simmer for 10 minutes to allow the flavours to infuse. Stir through the lemon juice and season with salt and pepper.

Meanwhile, to make the minted pea puree, bring a saucepan of salted water to the boil. Add the peas and cook for 3 minutes, or until tender. Drain, reserving 2½ tablespoons of cooking water. Combine the peas, mint, garlic and reserved cooking water in a food processor and process to a puree. With the motor running, pour in the olive oil in a slow, steady stream and process until combined. Season with salt and pepper. Set aside, keeping warm.

Heat a large ovenproof frying pan over high heat until very hot. Brush the trout fillets with the coconut oil or animal fat, season with salt and pepper and cook, skin-side down, for 30–60 seconds until crispy. Transfer the pan to the oven and cook the trout, still skin-side down, for 3½–4 minutes until the skin is golden and crisp (or cook to your liking). Flip the fillets, skin-side up, onto a plate and allow to rest for 2–3 minutes, keeping warm. At this point the trout will be perfectly cooked; slightly pink and moist in the middle.

To serve, stir the mint into the lemon broth, then ladle the hot broth into shallow serving bowls. Spoon in a good dollop of pea puree, then top with the trout.

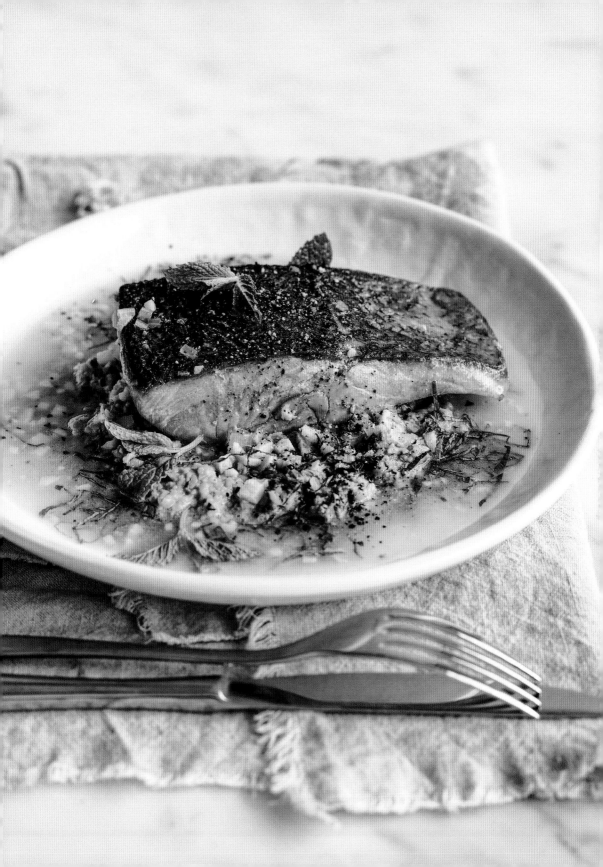

On a recent trip to Portugal, my wife, Nic, and I dined in a beautiful little place by the coast in Cascais. Portugal is one of the best countries in the world for pristine seafood, and this restaurant offered an array of wonderful fish. We chose the fried sardines and, wow, it was one of the most memorable dishes I have ever had. Here's my version of the recipe so you, too, can indulge in these cheap, plentiful and delicious morsels whenever you want.

SARDINES WITH LEMON AND AIOLI

Serves 2–4

15 whole sardines (about 600 g), gutted and backbones removed (ask your fishmonger)
100 g hemp or tapioca flour*
250 ml (1 cup) melted coconut oil or good-quality animal fat*
sea salt and freshly ground black pepper
150 g Aioli (page 165)
lemon wedges, to serve
smoked paprika, to serve

Marinade
4 garlic cloves, finely chopped
1 tablespoon chopped flat-leaf parsley leaves
1 tablespoon finely chopped oregano leaves
1½ teaspoons smoked paprika
zest and juice of 1 lemon
1 teaspoon ground cumin
1 long red chilli, deseeded and chopped
1 teaspoon sea salt

Chervil salad
1 large fennel bulb, finely sliced, fronds reserved
2 large handfuls of chervil leaves
zest and juice of 1 lemon
3 tablespoons olive oil

* See Glossary

To prepare the sardines, use kitchen scissors to snip any bones near the head. Rinse well under cold running water and pat dry with paper towel. Place the sardines in a large shallow bowl and set aside.

Place the marinade ingredients in a blender with 2 tablespoons of water and blend to a thick paste.

Rub the marinade over the sardines and toss well to completely coat. Cover and marinate in the fridge for 1 hour.

Working with one fish at a time, coat the sardines in the hemp or tapioca flour, shaking off any excess.

Heat the coconut oil or animal fat in a large, deep frying pan over medium heat. To test the heat, place a sardine in the pan. If the oil or fat immediately sizzles around the sardine, it is ready. Add the sardines in batches and cook for 30 seconds on each side, or until golden brown and cooked through. Remove the sardines with a slotted spoon and drain on paper towel. Season with salt and pepper, if desired.

To make the chervil salad, place the fennel, fennel fronds and chervil in a bowl. Add the lemon zest and juice and olive oil and gently toss. Season with salt and pepper.

Arrange the sardines on plates and serve with the aioli, chervil salad, lemon wedges and a sprinkling of smoked paprika.

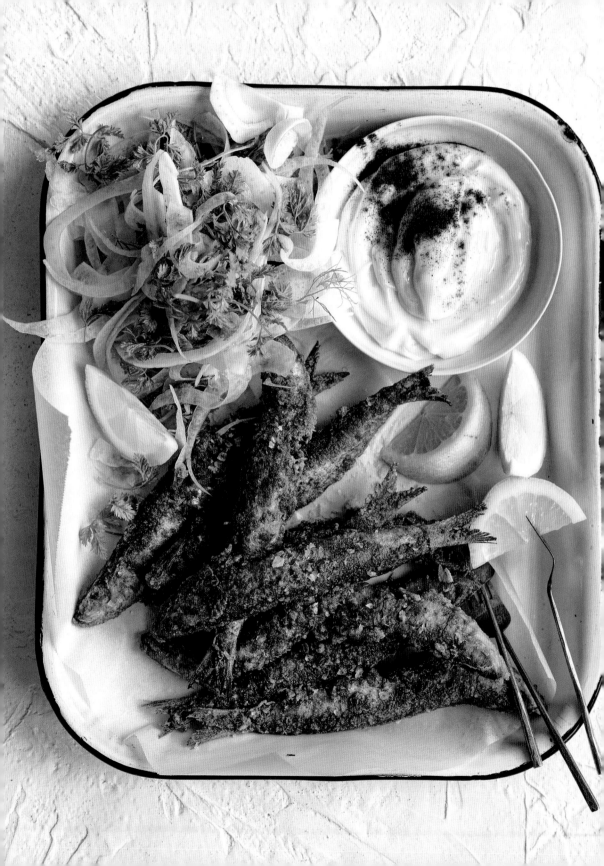

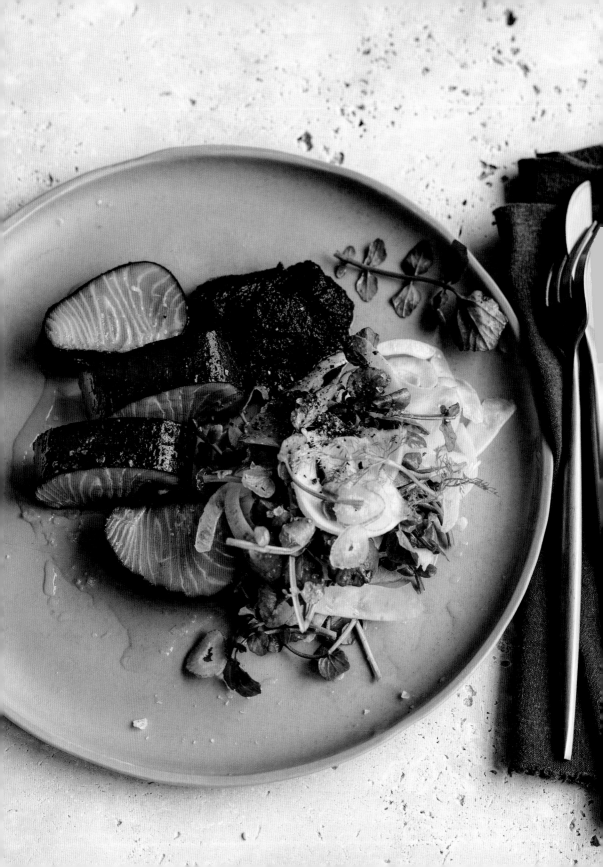

I am a huge fan of seaweed as it brings so much flavour and so many health benefits when consumed as part of a balanced diet. One of the best ways to enjoy it is to combine it with seafood, which makes sense as the two ingredients share the ocean together. This recipe is inspired by a dear friend of mine, Tetsuya Wakuda. I hope you love it as much as I have every time I have eaten it at his restaurant.

NORI-WRAPPED SALMON WITH BEETROOT HUMMUS

Serves 4

500 ml extra-virgin olive oil, plus extra if needed
2 star anise
2 teaspoons coriander seeds
1 lemon, sliced
4 x 140 g salmon fillets, skin removed
sea salt and freshly ground black pepper
4 nori* sheets

Beetroot hummus
500 g beetroot (about 2 large or 4 small)
3 tablespoons unhulled tahini
1 garlic clove, chopped
2 tablespoons extra-virgin olive oil
2 tablespoons lemon juice
1 tablespoon apple cider vinegar
2 teaspoons ground cumin
½ teaspoon sea salt

Fennel salad
2 tablespoons lemon juice
3 tablespoons olive oil
1 fennel bulb, finely sliced, fronds reserved
2 handfuls of watercress

* See Glossary

Preheat the oven to 180°C (160°C fan-forced). Line a baking tray with a wire rack.

To make the beetroot hummus, wrap the beetroot in foil and roast for 1½–2 hours until tender. Set aside to cool, then peel and roughly chop the beetroot and place in a food processor. Add the tahini, garlic, olive oil, lemon juice, vinegar, cumin and salt and process until smooth. Allow to cool.

Meanwhile, pour the olive oil into a saucepan pan large enough to fit the salmon fillets in a single layer. Place over very low heat, add the spices and lemon slices and warm the olive oil to 40–45°C. The oil should be warm to touch, not hot (see Note page 46).

Season the salmon fillets with salt and pepper. Place one salmon fillet on a nori sheet and roll over to wrap, allowing the nori sheet to overlap by 2 cm. Trim the ends off the nori sheet (save the trimmings to add to salads, or brush them with sesame oil and roast them to eat as a snack). Lightly brush the overlapping 2 cm of nori sheet with water and press to seal. Repeat with the remaining salmon fillets and nori sheets. Allow to stand for 2 minutes so the nori softens around the salmon.

Gently place the fillets in the pan, ensuring they are completely submerged in the warm oil (add more oil if not). Poach for 15–18 minutes until the flesh is tender and opaque. If you notice white dots leaching out on the surface of the fish (this is protein) and the flesh is turning a light pink, the oil is too hot, so you need to reduce the temperature.

Meanwhile, to make the salad, whisk the lemon juice and olive oil together in a small bowl and season to taste with salt and pepper. Combine the fennel and watercress in a large bowl, add the dressing and gently toss through to coat.

Carefully remove the salmon fillets with a spatula and transfer to the prepared tray to drain. Cut into thick slices.

Spoon the beetroot hummus onto serving plates, arrange the salmon and salad alongside and finish with a grind of pepper.

I tend to eat lighter meals in summer, which means more seafood and vegetables in my diet. It isn't a strict thing I do, I just listen to my body. So, when the warmer months come along, I love to whip up quick and easy dishes like this one, which can be on the table in a matter of minutes. You can swap out the trout for prawns or roast chicken or pork belly. Having said that, though, the trout is hard to beat.

TROUT, CAPERS AND ROCKET WITH ZUCCHINI NOODLES

Serves 4

1 whole hot-smoked rainbow trout (about 400 g), skin and bones removed and flesh flaked
3 tablespoons salted baby capers, rinsed and drained
2 large handfuls of rocket leaves, half left whole, half chopped
4 large zucchini (about 600 g), spiralised into thin noodles
chilli flakes, to serve
lemon wedges, to serve (optional)

Dressing
2 tablespoons Chilli Oil (page 169)
3 tablespoons garlic oil
3 tablespoons lemon juice
sea salt

To make the dressing, whisk the oils and lemon juice in a bowl and season with salt to taste.

Place the flaked trout flesh, capers, rocket and zucchini noodles in a bowl. Pour over the dressing and gently toss to coat. Serve immediately with a sprinkle of chilli flakes and the lemon wedges (if using).

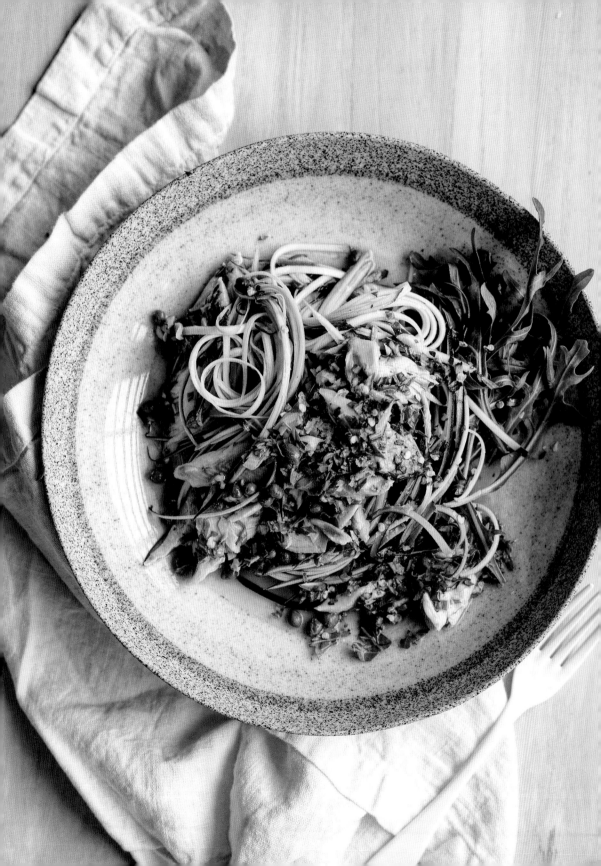

Fish and mushrooms is not a combination you see often, but it should be far more popular. The texture and flavour are so compatible. Sometimes I find eating fish can feel a little light, and that's where the mushrooms come in, adding a meatiness that really satiates. Here, I have used shiitake mushrooms as I truly love their flavour and the way they feel in the mouth. This is a dish that can be on the table in less than 20 minutes.

SNAPPER WITH SHIITAKE MUSHROOMS

Serves 4

2 tablespoons coconut oil or good-quality animal fat*
2 garlic cloves, finely chopped
1 tablespoon finely grated ginger
2 spring onions, finely chopped
200 g shiitake mushrooms, finely sliced
1 tablespoon apple cider vinegar
1 tablespoon tamari or coconut aminos*
1 teaspoon fish sauce, plus extra if needed
500 ml (2 cups) Fish or Brown Chicken Bone Broth (page 174 or 166)
4 x 160 g snapper fillets (or bream, mulloway, Spanish mackerel), skin on, each fillet halved
sea salt
1½ teaspoons sesame seeds, toasted
1 handful of coriander leaves
olive oil, to serve

* See Glossary

Heat the coconut oil or animal fat in a large frying pan over medium–high heat. Add the garlic, ginger and spring onion and sauté for 10 seconds. Stir in the shiitake mushroom and continue to sauté for 2 minutes, or until softened.

Pour the vinegar, tamari or coconut aminos and fish sauce into the pan and cook for 30 seconds, then pour in the broth. Bring to the boil, then reduce the heat to low, add the fish pieces, cover with the lid and simmer for 2½–3 minutes until the fish is cooked through. If needed, add a splash more fish sauce or a little salt for seasoning.

Sprinkle the sesame seeds and coriander over the snapper, drizzle with olive oil and serve.

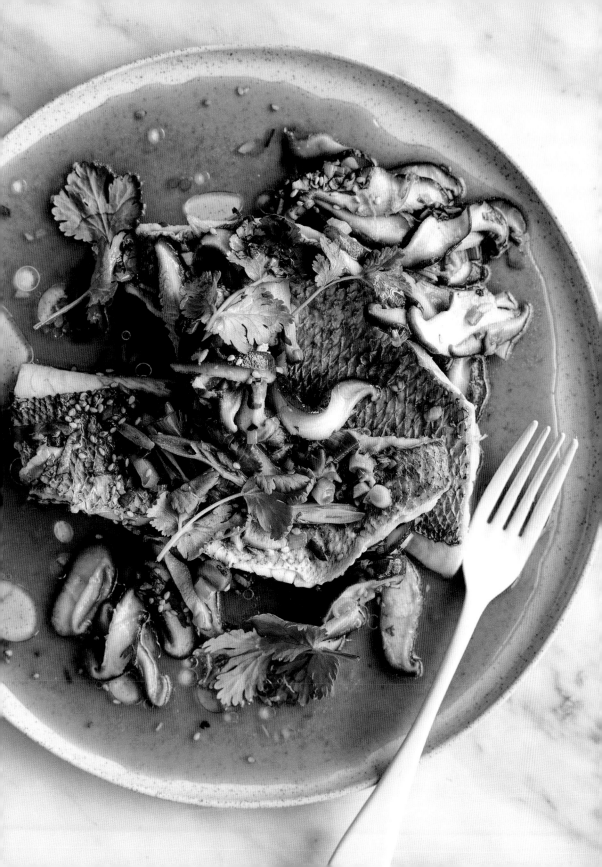

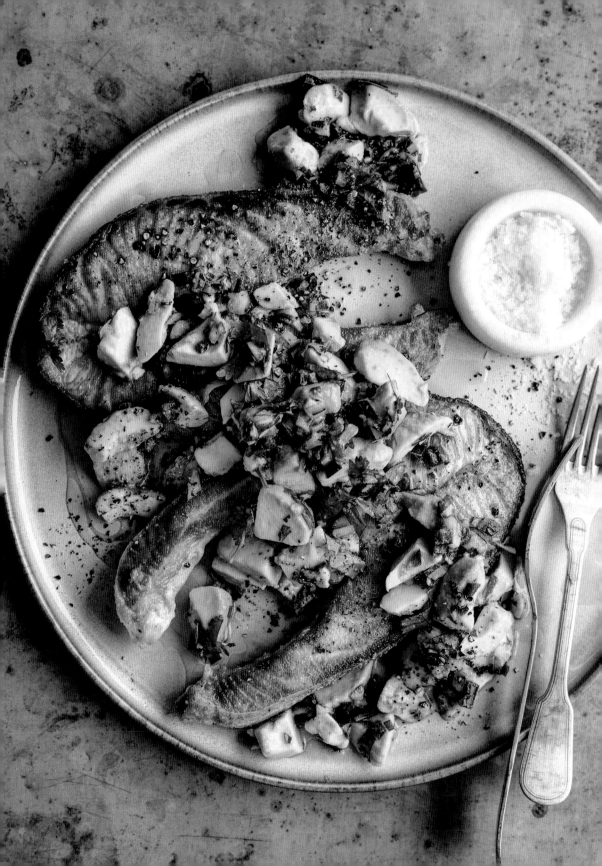

This is a combination I love to use in summer when avocados are cheap and abundant. My daughters enjoy making guacamole, so I can hand them the ingredients and they sort that out while I cook the fish. All up, dinner can be on the table in ten or so minutes, which is what all parents love. Thanks, girls xo.

SALMON CUTLETS WITH GUACAMOLE

Serves 2

2 x 230 g salmon cutlets
2 tablespoons coconut oil or
  good-quality animal fat*

Guacamole
2 avocados, diced
½ small red onion, finely chopped
1 long red chilli, finely chopped
1 tablespoon finely chopped
  coriander leaves
2 tablespoons lime juice,
  or to taste
3 tablespoons olive oil
sea salt and freshly ground
  black pepper

To serve (optional)
coriander sprigs
lime wedges

* See Glossary

Place all the guacamole ingredients in a bowl and mix to combine. Set aside.

Preheat a large frying pan over medium–high heat.

Brush the salmon with the coconut oil or animal fat, then season with salt and pepper. Cook for 2 minutes on each side, or until the flesh is tender and opaque (or cook to your liking). Allow to rest for 2 minutes.

Place the salmon on serving plates, spoon over the guacamole and serve with some coriander sprigs and lime wedges, if desired.

Sometimes the simple things in life are best. This is so true when it comes to a dish like this: the trout is the star and with a little support from the herbs you create a nice play of flavours for the tastebuds. The aim of poaching in olive oil is to cook the trout so gently that the flesh practically melts when a fork is pressed into it. Add a simple salad and a little lemon on the side and, voila, you have the perfect breakfast, lunch or dinner.

POACHED OCEAN TROUT WITH SOFT HERBS

Serves 4

500 ml (2 cups) extra-virgin olive oil, plus extra if needed and to serve
4 x 160 g ocean trout fillets, skin on
2 teaspoons finely grated lemon zest
1 teaspoon sea salt
2 handfuls of chervil leaves
2 handfuls of flat-leaf parsley leaves
1 handful of dill fronds
lemon wedges, to serve
Aioli (page 165), to serve
freshly ground black pepper

Place a wire rack in a baking tray.

Pour the olive oil into a saucepan large enough to fit the trout fillets in a single layer. Place over very low heat and warm the oil to 40–45°C. The oil should be warm to touch, not hot (see Note).

Meanwhile, rub the fillets with the lemon zest and salt.

Gently place the fillets in the pan, skin-side down, ensuring they are completely submerged in the warm oil (add more oil if not). Poach for 20 minutes, or until the flesh is deep pink and feels firm when lightly pressed. If you notice white dots on the surface (this is protein) and the flesh is turning pale pink, the oil is too hot, so you need to reduce the temperature. Carefully remove the fillets with a fish slice and transfer to the prepared tray to drain.

Serve the fillets with the chervil, parsley and dill on the side, lemon wedges for squeezing over the top, and the aioli. Drizzle over some extra oil and sprinkle with black pepper.

NOTE

It is best to sit the saucepan of oil on a rack so it is not directly touching the flame or hotplate. Use a thermometer to monitor the temperature – it should remain between 40 and 45°C at all times.

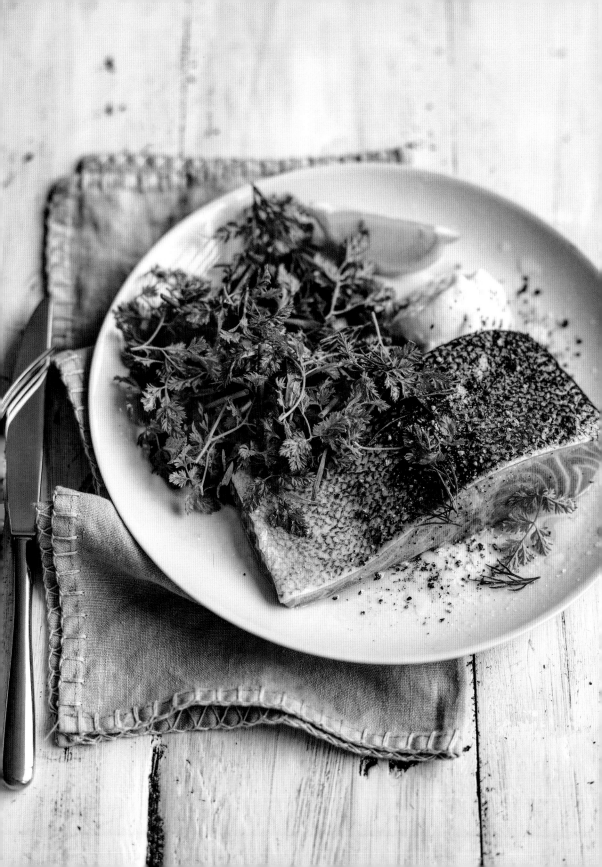

One of the recipes I have become quite famous for (well, on fishing trips to Darwin anyway) is my Singaporean chilli crab. And what an amazing dish it is. Still one of my all-time favourite meals to cook and eat, the crab does, however, require quite a bit of work. So, at home, when cooking crab for the family falls into the too-hard basket, we often have chilli mussels or prawns prepared exactly the same way, with the same delicious sauce, a lot less mess and just the same outcome – smiles all round. Try this sauce with any seafood you can get your hands on.

CHILLI MUSSELS

Serves 2

1 tablespoon coconut oil or
good-quality animal fat*
8 garlic cloves, chopped
3 bird's eye chillies, deseeded
and chopped
4 cm piece of ginger, cut into
matchsticks
2 tablespoons finely chopped
coriander roots
275 ml Fish Bone Broth
(page 174)
125 ml (½ cup) Hoisin Sauce
(page 174)
2 tablespoons fish sauce
250 g cherry tomatoes, halved
1 kg mussels, scrubbed and
debearded
3 spring onions, green part
only, chopped
1 handful of mixed mint,
Vietnamese mint and
coriander leaves

Sweet chilli sauce
125 ml (½ cup) coconut vinegar
115 g (⅓ cup) honey
2 tablespoons fish sauce
4 garlic cloves, peeled
4 cm piece of ginger,
finely chopped
3 long red chillies, chopped
1 tablespoon tapioca flour*,
mixed with 2 tablespoons water

* See Glossary

To make the sweet chilli sauce, place the coconut vinegar, honey, fish sauce, garlic, ginger, chilli and 125 ml (½ cup) of water in a food processor and blend to a paste. Pour into a saucepan and bring to the boil. Turn down the heat to low and simmer for about 5 minutes until the sauce has reduced by half. Whisk in the tapioca mixture and continue to whisk for 30 seconds. Remove from the heat and cool.

Heat the coconut oil or animal fat in a wok or large saucepan over medium–high heat. Add the garlic, chilli, ginger and coriander root and cook for about 2 minutes until fragrant. Add the sweet chilli sauce, broth, hoisin sauce and fish sauce, stir well and bring to the boil. Cover and simmer for 5 minutes. Stir in the tomato halves and cook for 3 minutes.

Add the mussels to the wok or pan, cover with a lid and cook for 3–4 minutes until the mussels open. Holding down the lid, shake the pan to redistribute the mussels. Discard any mussels that do not open. Scatter over the spring onion and mixed herbs and serve.

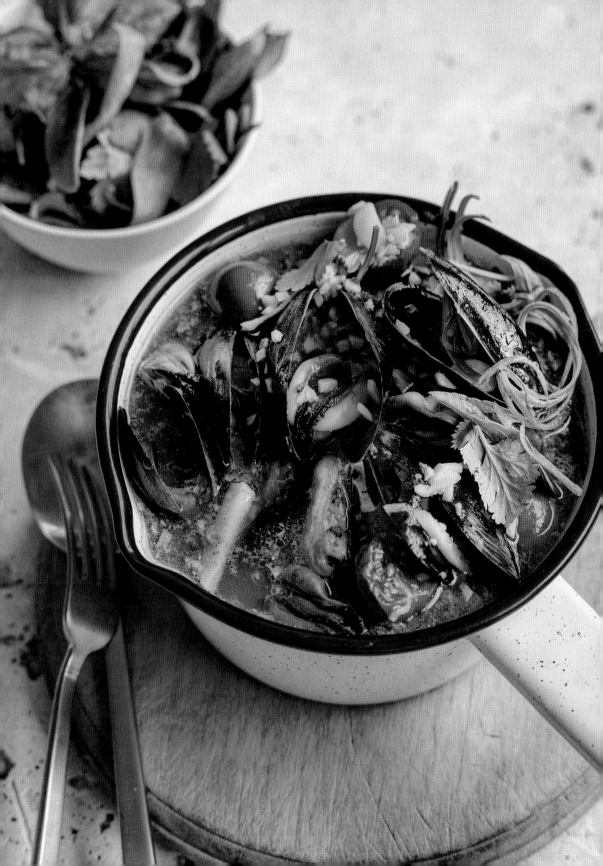

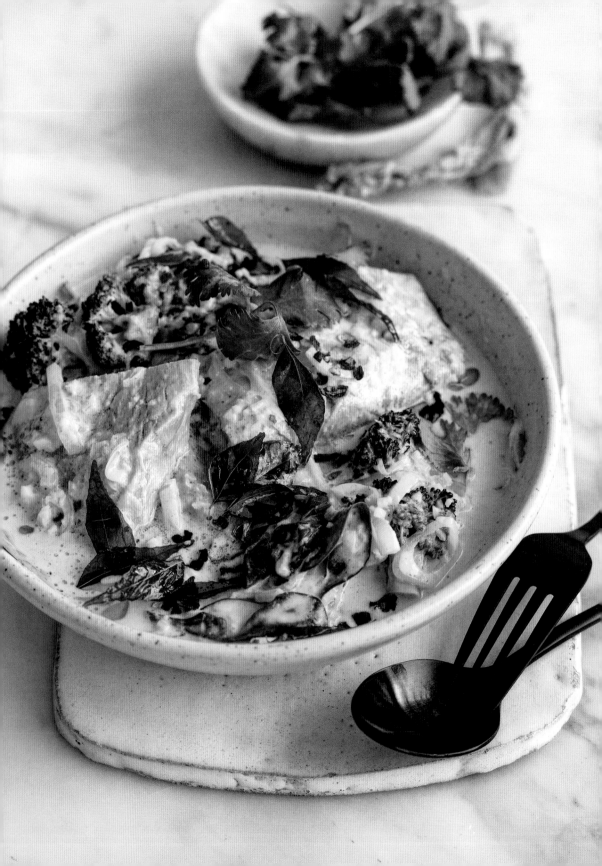

I am a big fan of curries. Making a curry from scratch can be therapeutic and fun to do, especially if you have kids who don't mind using a mortar and pestle.

WILD SALMON CURRY

Serves 4

80 ml (⅓ cup) melted coconut
   oil or good-quality animal fat*,
   plus extra for greasing
2 teaspoons ground turmeric
2 teaspoons ground coriander
1 teaspoon ground cumin
1 head of broccoli, broken
   into florets
sea salt and freshly ground
   black pepper
4 x 180 g salmon fillets, skin on
   or off, pin-boned
1 tablespoon lime juice
1 onion, sliced
2.5 cm piece of ginger,
   finely grated
4 garlic cloves, finely chopped
5 cardamom pods, crushed
1 cinnamon stick
1 teaspoon chilli flakes
12 fresh curry leaves
400 ml coconut cream
140 ml Fish Bone Broth
   (page 174) or water
1 large handful of baby
   spinach leaves
1 handful of coriander leaves
Cauliflower Rice (page 167),
   to serve (optional)
lime cheeks, to serve (optional)

* See Glossary

Preheat the oven to 200°C (180°C fan-forced). Lightly grease a baking tray with coconut oil or animal fat.

Mix the ground spices in a small bowl and set aside.

Place the broccoli florets, 1 tablespoon of the oil or fat and half the spice mixture in a bowl and toss to coat well. Transfer to the prepared tray, spread out in a single layer and season with a little salt. Roast for 15 minutes, or until the broccoli is golden. Set aside.

Rub the remaining spice mixture into the flesh of the salmon fillets, season with salt and pepper and pour over half the lime juice. Cover and marinate in the fridge for 10 minutes.

Meanwhile, heat the remaining oil or fat in a large frying pan over medium heat. Add the onion and sauté for 5 minutes, or until softened. Add the ginger and garlic and sauté for a further 30 seconds, then stir in the cardamom pods, cinnamon stick, chilli flakes, curry leaves and a pinch of pepper and cook for 1 minute.

Add the roasted broccoli, coconut cream and broth or water to the pan and mix to combine. Place the salmon, flesh-side down, in the pan, cover with the lid and poach for 6 minutes, or until the fish is almost cooked through. Add the spinach and gently stir through.

Season the salmon curry with salt and pepper, pour over the remaining lime juice and scatter on the coriander leaves. Serve with the cauliflower rice and lime cheeks, if desired.

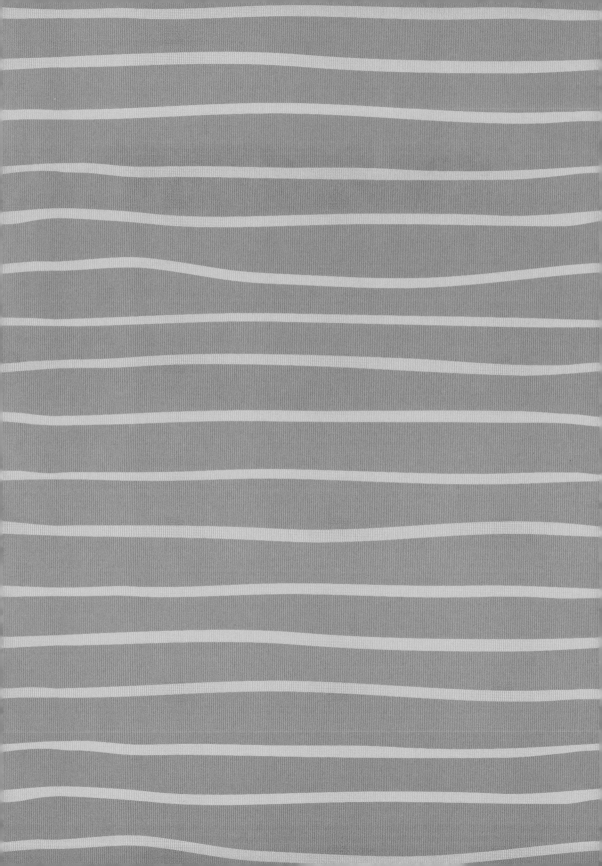

CHICKEN
& DUCK

Chicken is the most popular meat consumed in Australia. From an ethical consideration, I would rather get my protein from pasture-raised cattle as only one animal loses its life to supply a lot more meat for a lot more of us. In saying that, do I eat and enjoy chicken? You bet! Here is a delicious chicken burger recipe inspired by my travels in Portugal.

PIRI-PIRI CHICKEN BURGERS

Serves 4

1 tablespoon coconut oil or good-quality animal fat*, plus extra for brushing
½ onion, finely diced
2 garlic cloves, finely chopped
1 teaspoon chopped thyme leaves
600 g chicken mince
1 egg
zest of 1 lemon
1 teaspoon sea salt
½ teaspoon freshly ground black pepper
1 lemon, halved, to serve

Piri-piri sauce
2 tablespoons coconut oil or good-quality animal fat*
1 tablespoon sweet paprika
1½ teaspoons ground cumin
1½ teaspoons ground coriander
1 red capsicum, deseeded and chopped
½ onion, chopped
3 garlic cloves, chopped
4 long red chillies, deseeded and roughly chopped (leave the seeds in if you like it hot)
1 teaspoon grated ginger
3½ tablespoons lemon juice
100 ml olive oil
sea salt and freshly ground black pepper

* See Glossary

To make the piri-piri sauce, combine the coconut oil or animal fat, paprika and ground spices in a frying pan over medium heat and cook for 10 seconds until fragrant. Add the capsicum, onion, garlic, chilli and ginger and cook for 5 minutes, or until the onion is softened. Add 180 ml (¾ cup) of water, stir through the vegetables and bring to the boil. Reduce the heat to low, then simmer for 10 minutes until the sauce has thickened and reduced by three-quarters. Allow to cool, then add the lemon juice, transfer the mixture to a blender and blend until smooth. With the motor running, pour in the olive oil in a slow, steady stream and blend until incorporated. Season with salt and pepper and set aside to cool.

To start on the chicken burgers, heat the coconut oil or animal fat in a frying pan over medium heat. Add the onion and sauté for 5 minutes, or until softened. Stir in the garlic and thyme and cook for 30 seconds, or until fragrant. Remove from the heat and allow to cool. Place the cooled onion mixture in a bowl and add the mince, egg and lemon zest. Add the salt and pepper and mix well. Shape into eight or nine patties.

Heat a barbecue grill to medium–hot or a chargrill pan over medium–high heat. Brush with a little extra oil or fat, add the patties and cook for 4 minutes. Turn the patties and continue to cook for 2–3 minutes until they are charred and cooked through.

Arrange the burgers on a platter and spoon over the piri-piri sauce. Serve with the lemon halves for squeezing over the top.

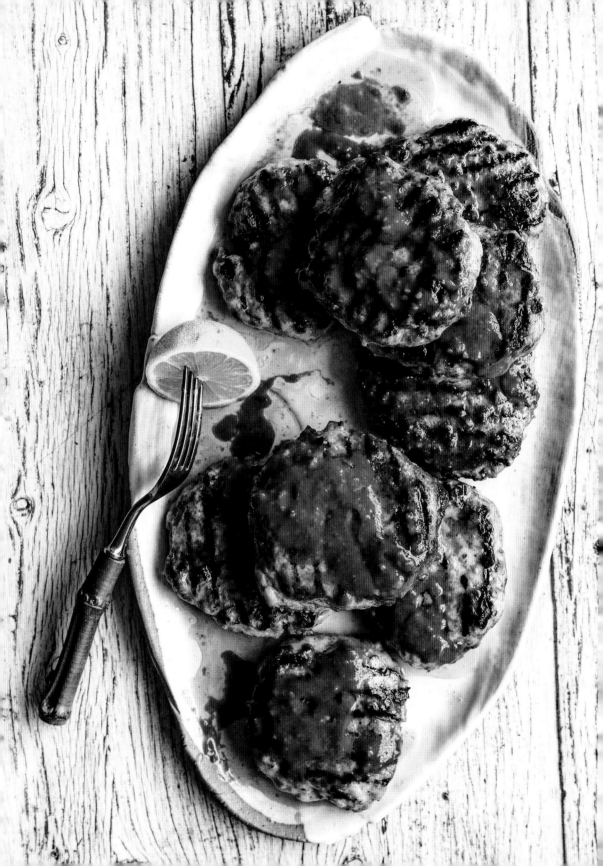

Poaching chicken breast, a technique many cultures employ, is a very simple way to ensure the flesh stays juicy and moist. I love the South-East Asian take, where poaching the chicken in coconut milk or cream helps it to soak up all that delicious fatty flavour and brings to life the blandest part of the chicken. Turn this into a meal by simply adding some veg or salad.

COCONUT-POACHED CHICKEN BREAST

Serves 4

4 chicken breasts
sea salt
600 ml Brown Chicken Bone
   Broth page 166)
1–2 long red chillies, finely sliced
   (depending on how hot you
   like it)
2 lemongrass stems, pale part
   only, finely sliced
2 makrut lime leaves*
1 tablespoon finely grated ginger
800 ml coconut milk
1 tablespoon fish sauce,
   plus extra if needed
1 tablespoon lime juice
1 bunch of Chinese broccoli
   (gai lan), trimmed and cut
   into thirds

To serve
Cauliflower Rice (page 167)
1 handful of coriander leaves
1 handful of Thai basil leaves
a few drops of sesame oil
lime wedges

* See Glossary

Season the chicken breasts with salt and stand for 15 minutes to come to room temperature.

Meanwhile, combine the broth, half the chilli, the lemongrass, makrut lime leaves and ginger in a large saucepan and bring to a gentle simmer over medium heat. Simmer for 20 minutes to allow the flavours to develop. Stir in the coconut milk and fish sauce and bring back to a simmer.

Reduce the heat to medium–low, add the chicken to the pan, making sure it is submerged in the coconut broth, and poach for about 20 minutes until it is cooked through. Remove the chicken from the pan and rest for 5 minutes, keeping warm, before slicing.

Mix the lime juice into the coconut broth and check for seasoning, adding more fish sauce or salt if needed.

Meanwhile, bring a saucepan of salted water to the boil. Add the Chinese broccoli and cook for 3–4 minutes until tender. Drain and set aside.

To serve, divide the cauliflower rice among serving bowls, arrange the chicken on top, then ladle over the coconut broth. Add the Chinese broccoli, sprinkle over the remaining chilli, the coriander and Thai basil and drizzle over the sesame oil. Serve with the lime wedges on the side.

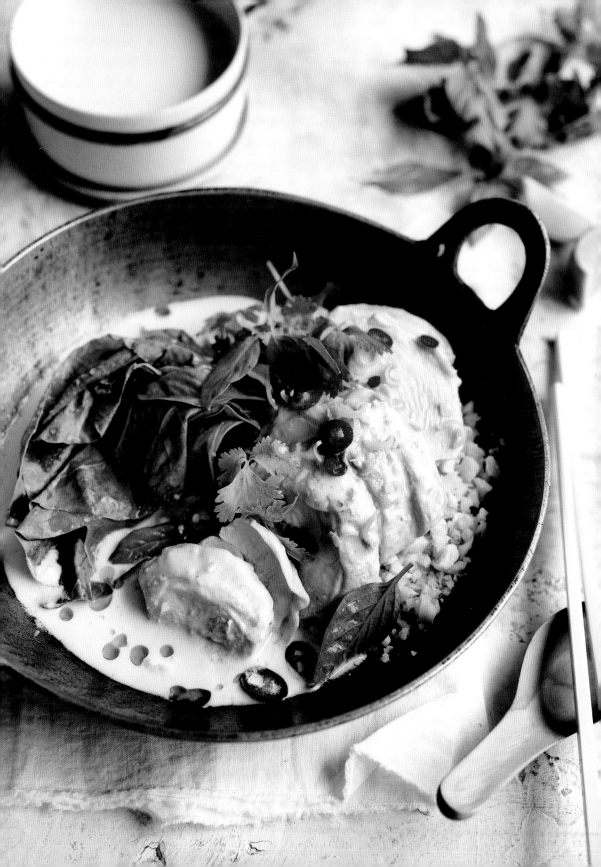

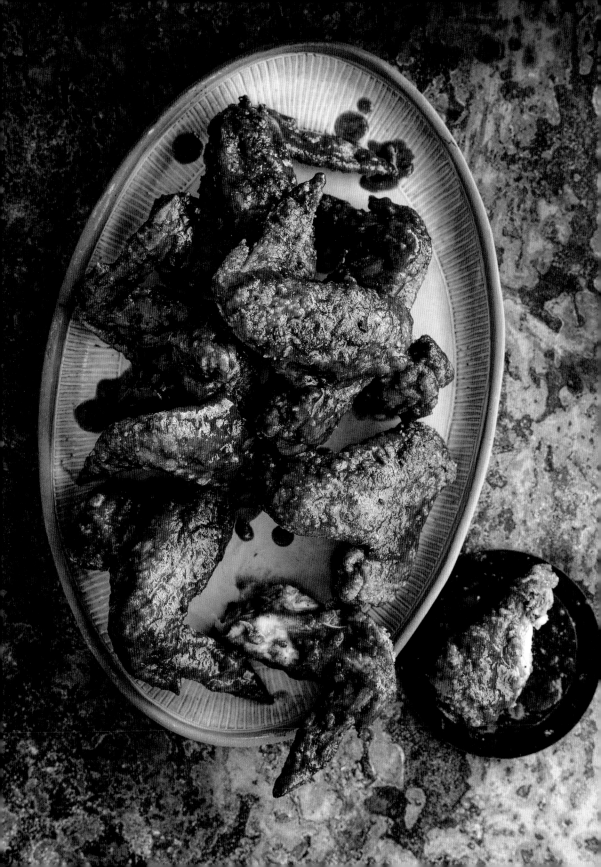

If you are like me, you have probably wondered why buffalo wings are so named. (When I first heard of them, I pictured a buffalo with wings!) Well, I went digging to find out more about these delicious spicy chicken morsels and, apparently, the name comes from the town of Buffalo in New York, where they were first created. So, now we have that out of the way, let's get into the real delight of creating these wings at home.

BUFFALO WINGS

Serves 4

1.2 kg chicken wings
coconut oil, for deep-frying
120 g tapioca flour*
sea salt and freshly ground
  black pepper
150 ml Hot Sauce (page 174)

Marinade
80 ml (⅓ cup) melted Smoked
  Lard (page 176) or duck fat
1 teaspoon ground cumin
1 teaspoon garlic powder
1 teaspoon onion powder
2 teaspoons finely grated ginger
1 tablespoon smoked paprika
1 tablespoon honey
1½ tablespoons apple cider
  vinegar
½ teaspoon fine sea salt
1 pinch of freshly ground
  black pepper

* See Glossary

Combine the marinade ingredients in a large bowl and whisk together well.

Toss the wings in the marinade and turn to coat well. Cover and marinate in the fridge for 2 hours or, for best results, overnight.

Heat the coconut oil in a wok or large saucepan to 160°C. (To test, drop a small piece of chicken into the oil – if it starts to bubble around the chicken immediately, the oil is ready.)

Place the tapioca flour in a shallow bowl and season with salt and pepper. One at a time, add the chicken wings, turn to coat and shake well to dust off any excess flour.

Carefully add the wings in batches to the hot oil and deep-fry for 6–6½ minutes until cooked through and golden. Remove with a slotted spoon and place on paper towel to drain. Season with salt and pepper.

Transfer the wings to a bowl, pour over the hot sauce and toss the chicken to evenly coat.

Arrange the buffalo wings on a platter and serve.

Roast chicken is, without a doubt, one of my all-time favourite dishes to cook at home. I reckon I have cooked it hundreds of times – and each time a little differently; whether it's the spices I use, or the stuffing I choose, or the sauce I prepare to accompany it. The beautiful thing about a good ol' roast chook is that it is so, so simple. Here, I have butterflied the chicken, to speed up the cooking process, and served it with a delicious herb sauce that the whole family will enjoy.

BUTTERFLIED CHICKEN WITH HERB SAUCE

Serves 6

8 garlic cloves, peeled
3 tablespoons lemon juice
½ teaspoon cayenne pepper
1 teaspoon ground cumin
1 pinch of saffron threads
  (about 20)
80 ml (⅓ cup) melted ghee
  or good-quality animal fat*,
  plus extra for brushing
sea salt and freshly ground
  black pepper
1 x 1.8 kg chicken, butterflied
  with breastbone in (ask your
  butcher)

Herb sauce
3 tablespoons tarragon leaves
3 tablespoons dill fronds
3 tablespoons flat-leaf
  parsley leaves
250 ml (1 cup) olive oil
1 tablespoon lemon juice,
  or to taste

* See Glossary

Preheat the oven to 200°C (180°C fan-forced).

Place the garlic, lemon juice, cayenne pepper, cumin, saffron and ghee or fat in a blender and blend to a smooth paste. Season with salt and pepper.

Pat the chicken dry with paper towel. Evenly cover the entire bird with the garlic paste. Cover and marinate in the fridge for 30 minutes.

Heat a large frying pan over medium–high heat and brush with some ghee or fat. Cook the chicken (reserve the marinade) for 2–3 minutes on each side until nicely golden.

Transfer the chicken to a roasting tin, pour over the pan juices and the reserved marinade and roast, basting occasionally with the juices in the tin, for 25 minutes. Loosely cover the tin with foil and roast for a further 15–20 minutes until the chicken is golden and the juices run clear when the thigh is pierced with a skewer. Place the chicken on a platter and allow to rest for 5 minutes, keeping warm. Season with extra salt and pepper if needed.

Meanwhile, place all the herb sauce ingredients in a food processor and blend to a chunky sauce. Season with salt and pepper to taste and add extra lemon juice if desired.

To serve, cut the chicken into portions and drizzle over the herb sauce.

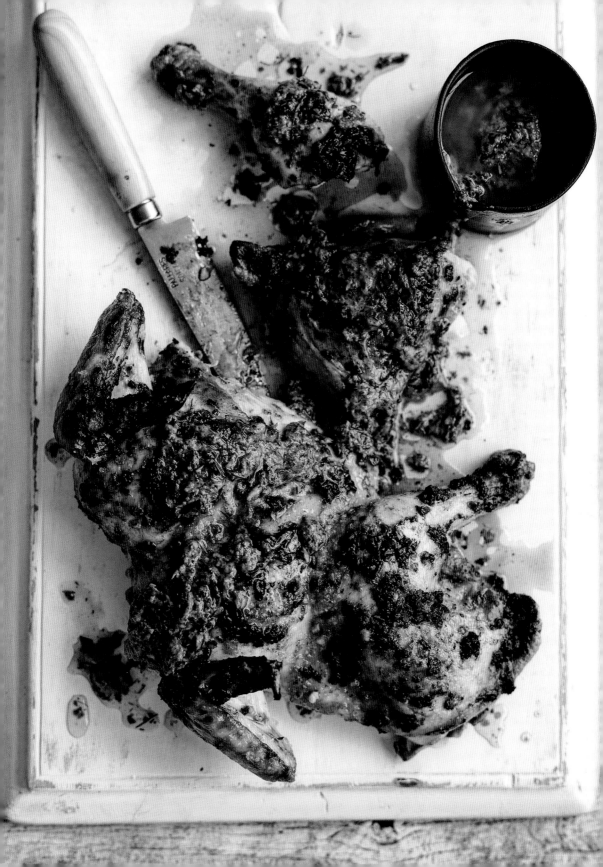

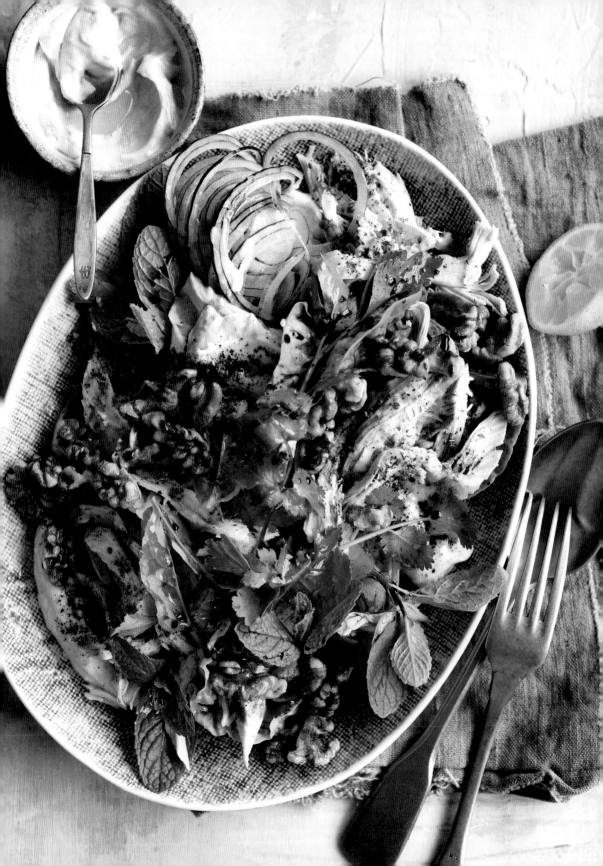

Tarator is one of the tastiest and easiest sauces you will ever make. Originating in the Middle East, the tahini base is balanced out with lemon juice, garlic and cumin. It works well as a replacement for mayonnaise and is delicious served with any roasted or grilled meats, seafood, vegetables and even eggs. In this recipe, the tarator sauce enhances and binds the roast chicken with a wonderful salad of walnuts, onion and herbs to create a glorious lunch or dinner. You can add some boiled eggs for an extra kick of fat and protein, if you like.

CHICKEN TARATOR SALAD

Serves 4–6

600 g leftover roast chicken
  breast and thigh, shredded
1 lemon, halved

Tarator sauce
300 g coconut yoghurt
3 tablespoons hulled tahini
3 tablespoons lemon juice
1½ teaspoons ground cumin
1 garlic clove, finely grated
sea salt and freshly ground
  black pepper

Salad
80 ml (⅓ cup) extra-virgin
  olive oil
3 tablespoons lemon juice
1½ teaspoons sumac, plus extra
  to serve
1 cos lettuce (or 2 baby cos),
  shredded
2 handfuls of coriander leaves
2 handfuls of mint leaves
2 handfuls of flat-leaf
  parsley leaves
1 small red onion, finely sliced
150 g walnuts, toasted and
  chopped, plus extra to serve

Place all the tarator sauce ingredients in a blender, add 2 tablespoons of water and blend until smooth and creamy. Taste and season with more salt and pepper if needed. Add a little more water if you prefer a thinner sauce.

To make the salad, whisk the olive oil, lemon juice and sumac in a small bowl and season with salt and pepper. Place the remaining salad ingredients in a large bowl, pour over half the dressing and gently toss to combine. Season with more salt and pepper if needed.

Smear half the tarator sauce on a platter, arrange the salad and shredded chicken on top and drizzle on the remaining dressing. Scatter over the extra walnuts, sprinkle on the extra sumac and serve with the lemon and the remaining tarator sauce.

Duck, with its skin on and its unctuous flesh, is one of my favourite meats to consume, as it can handle big, bold flavours. This red curry is the perfect vehicle to bring duck and pineapple together in one tantalising bowl.

RED CURRY OF DUCK WITH PINEAPPLE

Serves 4

1 x 2 kg duck
sea salt and freshly ground
   black pepper
4 spring onions, 3 cut into 4 cm
   batons, white part and green
   parts separated; 1 left whole
1 lime, halved
1 tablespoon coconut oil or
   good-quality animal fat*
100 g red curry paste
600 ml coconut cream
300 ml Brown Chicken Bone
   Broth (page 166)
2 makrut lime leaves*
1 head of broccoli, cut into florets
200 g pineapple, cut into
   2 cm pieces
fish sauce, to taste

To serve
1 handful of Thai basil leaves
Crispy Shallots (page 172)
Cauliflower Rice (page 167)

* See Glossary

Preheat the oven to 210°C (190°C fan-forced). Place a wire rack in a large roasting tin.

Rinse the duck and pat dry with paper towel. Season generously inside and out with salt and pepper. Using a skewer, prick the skin on each duck breast about ten times (this helps render the fat while roasting). Place the bird in the prepared tin, stuff the whole spring onion and a lime half into the cavity and set aside for 40 minutes to come to room temperature.

Next, transfer the duck to the oven and roast for 40 minutes. Drain off the fat in the tin (reserve for another use) and any juices, then return to the oven for a further 50 minutes until the duck is cooked. Loosely cover and rest in a warm place for 20 minutes.

When the duck is cool enough to handle, use a sharp knife to remove the breast and legs. Shred any flesh remaining on the carcass (discard the carcass). Slice the breast into pieces and keep the legs whole. (If you prefer, shred the meat off the legs and discard the bones.)

Melt the coconut oil or animal fat in a large saucepan over medium heat. Add the spring onion whites and stir-fry for 1 minute, or until starting to colour. Add the curry paste and cook for 30 seconds, or until fragrant. Gradually stir in the coconut cream and broth, then add the makrut lime leaves and bring to a simmer. Add the broccoli and cook for 10 minutes, then add the pineapple and cook for 15 minutes, or until the broccoli is tender and the sauce is reduced to a pouring cream consistency. Stir in the shredded duck and the remaining spring onion and cook for 3 minutes, or until heated through. Remove from the heat.

Squeeze a little juice from the remaining lime half into the curry, taste and season with some fish sauce and salt. Ladle the curry into serving bowls and sprinkle on the Thai basil and crispy shallots. Serve with the cauliflower rice.

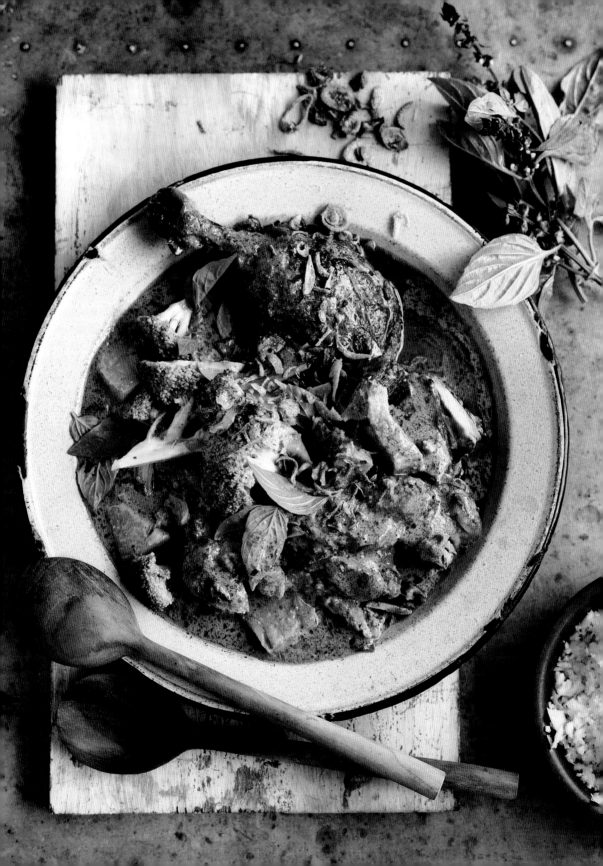

This recipe is a real show stopper. If you want to break out of ketosis, simply up your healthy carbs, as this recipe does, by using pumpkin. If you want to go lower carb and stay purely keto, replace the pumpkin with zucchini or serve in lettuce cups.

MEXICAN CHICKEN WITH ROASTED PUMPKIN AND AVOCADO AND TOMATO SALSA

HIGH-CARB DAY

Serves 4

1 butternut pumpkin (1.8–2 kg), halved lengthways, deseeded
2 tablespoons coconut oil or good-quality animal fat*, melted
sea salt and freshly ground black pepper
1 spring onion, finely sliced
1 handful of coriander leaves
3 tablespoons sliced pickled jalapeno chilli
lime cheeks, to serve

Mexican chicken

2 tablespoons coconut oil or good-quality animal fat*
2 onions, finely chopped
2 garlic cloves, finely chopped
1 tablespoon chipotle chillies in adobo sauce, chopped, plus extra if desired
700 g boneless chicken thighs, skin off, cut into 1 cm thick strips
1 teaspoon smoked paprika, plus extra to serve
1 teaspoon ground cumin
½ teaspoon ground coriander
1½ tablespoons tomato paste
400 g whole peeled tomatoes, crushed (see Note)
150 ml Brown Chicken Bone Broth (page 166) or water

Avocado and tomato salsa

1 avocado, sliced
2 tomatoes, deseeded and cut into 1 cm dice
¼ red onion, finely chopped
1 long red chilli, deseeded and finely chopped
2 tablespoons lime juice
2 tablespoons extra-virgin olive oil

* See Glossary

Preheat the oven to 180°C (160°C fan-forced).

Brush the pumpkin with the coconut oil or animal fat. Place, cut-side up, in a roasting tin and sprinkle with salt and pepper. Roast for 1¼–1½ hours until tender.

Meanwhile, to make the Mexican chicken, heat the coconut oil or animal fat in a large frying pan over medium–high heat. Add the onion and cook for 5 minutes, or until softened. Stir in the garlic and chipotle chilli and cook for 1 minute, or until fragrant. Add the chicken and sauté for 5 minutes, or until browned. Add the spices and tomato paste and cook for 1 minute, then mix in the tomatoes and broth. Reduce the heat to medium–low and simmer for 15 minutes, or until the chicken is cooked through and the sauce has thickened. Season with salt and pepper. If you like things a little spicier, add some extra chipotle chilli.

Mix the avocado and tomato salsa ingredients in a bowl and season with salt and pepper.

Carefully transfer the roasted pumpkin to two serving plates. Spoon over the Mexican chicken, then top with the avocado and tomato salsa. Finish with a sprinkle of spring onion, coriander, jalapeno chilli and a pinch of smoked paprika and serve with the lime cheeks.

NOTE

I prefer to buy diced and whole peeled tomatoes in jars rather than cans, due to the presence of Bisphenol A (BPA) in some cans. BPA is a toxic chemical that can interfere with our hormonal system.

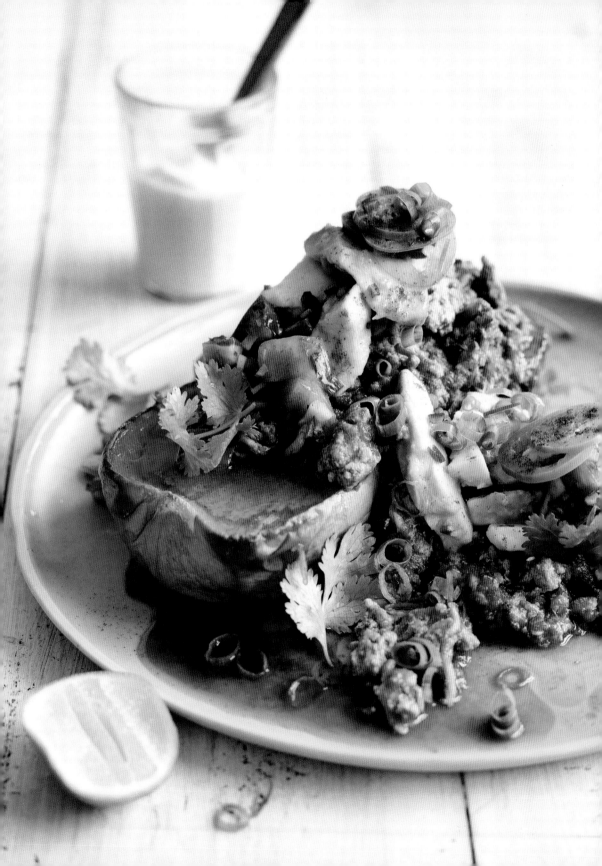

Travelling through Malaysia, my go-to dish is always Hainanese chicken rice – these days without the rice. The sheer beauty of this dish is the poached chicken, and its luxurious melt-in-the-mouth texture, with the gut-healthy chicken broth. I recommend making extra because the chicken cold the next day, either plain or in a salad, is sensational.

HAINANESE CHICKEN

Serves 6

1 x 1.8 kg chicken
sea salt
3 spring onions, white part cut into 5 cm batons, green part finely sliced on an angle
2.5 cm piece of ginger, cut into matchsticks
3.7 litres Brown Chicken Bone Broth (page 166), plus extra if needed
2 tablespoons coconut oil or good-quality animal fat*
2 French shallots, finely chopped
3 garlic cloves, finely chopped
500 g Cauliflower and Broccoli Rice (page 167)
3 baby bok choy, trimmed
1 Lebanese cucumber, cut into 4 cm lengths

Tamari and ginger dressing
80 ml (⅓ cup) tamari or coconut aminos*
3 cm piece of ginger, cut into matchsticks
1 teaspoon sesame oil

Chilli sauce
3 tablespoons Fermented Chilli Sambal (page 172)
1 tablespoon olive oil
1 tablespoon lime juice

* See Glossary

Rinse the chicken and pat dry with paper towel. Season generously inside and out with 3 teaspoons of salt. Place on a plate and stand for 40 minutes to come to room temperature.

Place the spring onion whites, ginger and broth in a stockpot and bring to the boil over medium–high heat. Carefully add the chicken, making sure it is fully submerged in the broth (add extra broth or water if needed). Bring the broth back to the boil, cover with the lid, then reduce the heat to medium–low and simmer for 15 minutes. Turn off the heat and allow the chicken to poach, undisturbed, for 45 minutes, or until the chicken is cooked through. To check, insert a skewer in the thigh; if the juices run clear, the chicken is cooked. Remove the chicken from the broth, reserving the broth. Allow the chicken to rest for 10 minutes, keeping warm.

Meanwhile, heat the coconut oil or animal fat in a large frying pan over medium heat. Add the shallot and sauté for 5 minutes, or until softened. Add the garlic and sauté for 30 seconds, or until fragrant. Stir in the cauliflower and broccoli rice and cook, stirring frequently, for 3 minutes, or until just warmed through. Season with a little salt.

To make the tamari and ginger dressing, pour 100 ml of the reserved broth into a small saucepan. Add the tamari or coconut aminos, ginger and sesame oil, place over medium–low heat and simmer for 10 minutes, or until the ginger is softened. Set aside.

Bring the pot of broth back to the boil and simmer until reduced by half (roughly 1.5 litres). Reduce the heat to medium–low, add the bok choy and simmer until wilted. Add the spring onion greens and simmer for 1 minute. Season with salt and pepper if needed.

Mix the chilli sauce ingredients in a bowl. Set aside.

Cut the chicken into large pieces Chinese-style, using a cleaver to cut through the bone. Divide the broccoli and cauliflower rice among serving bowls, then add the bok choy and chicken. Pour over some broth, spoon the tamari and ginger dressing over the chicken, add the cucumber and serve with the chilli sauce.

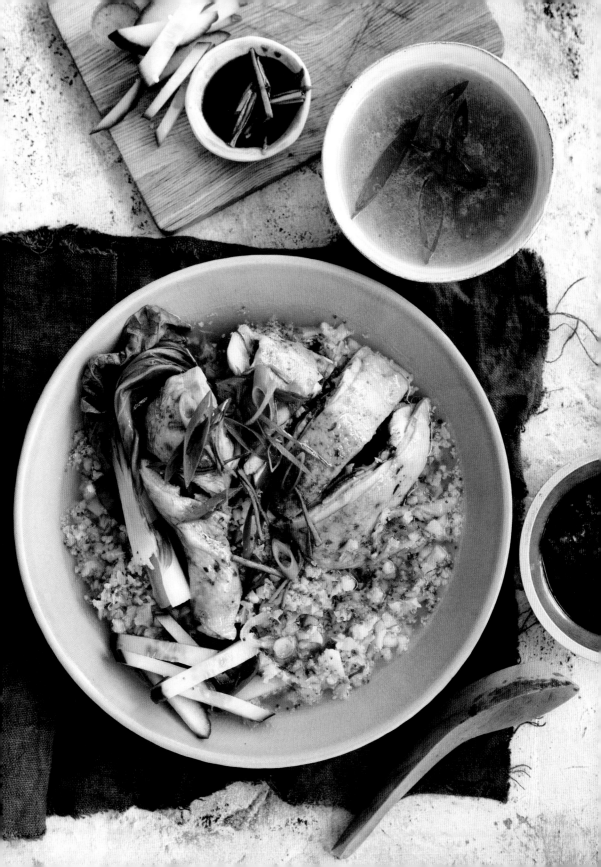

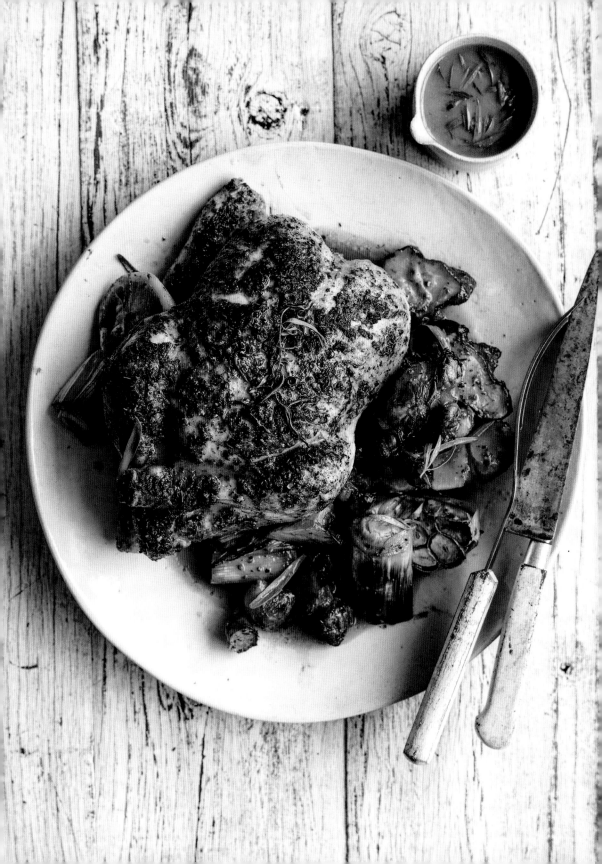

Tarragon, an often-overlooked herb, adds a beautiful flavour to many dishes. We grow it at home in the garden as it's a real staple for us. This recipe is a glorious way to show off its wondrous qualities – it turns the humble roast chook into one of the most memorable meals ever. This is in my top ten for home-cooked roasts.

ROAST CHICKEN WITH TARRAGON JUS   HIGH-CARB DAY

Serves 4

2 garlic bulbs, halved horizontally
1 onion, thickly sliced
400 g Jerusalem artichokes,
　scrubbed and thickly sliced
2 leeks, white part only, cut into
　3 cm lengths
1 x 1.8 kg chicken
3 tablespoons coconut oil or
　good-quality animal fat*, melted
2½ tablespoons Cajun spice
sea salt and freshly ground
　black pepper
1 lemon, halved
250 ml (1 cup) Brown Chicken
　Bone Broth (page 166)

Tarragon Jus
400 ml Chicken Jus (page 167)
3 tablespoons tarragon leaves

* See Glossary

Preheat the oven to 200°C (180°C fan-forced).

Scatter the garlic and onion over the base of a large roasting tin, then arrange the Jerusalem artichoke and leek on top.

Rinse the chicken and pat dry with paper towel. Rub with the coconut oil or animal fat, sprinkle over the Cajun spice and season generously inside and out with salt and pepper. Stuff a lemon half into the cavity, then tie the legs together with kitchen string. Place the chicken in the tin, squeeze over the juice from the remaining lemon half and pour the broth around the chicken.

Roast the chicken, basting occasionally with the juices in the tin, for 30 minutes. Reduce the temperature to 180°C (160°C fan-forced) and roast for a further 45–55 minutes until the chicken is golden and the juices run clear when the thigh is pierced with a skewer. Cover the skin with baking paper if it starts to darken too much during cooking.

Remove the chicken from the tin, cover loosely and rest in a warm place for 10 minutes.

Meanwhile, to make the tarragon jus, place the chicken jus and tarragon in a small saucepan and bring to a simmer over medium heat. Simmer for 5 minutes to allow the flavours to infuse. If needed, season with a little salt and pepper.

Serve the chicken with the garlic, onion, Jerusalem artichoke, leek and tarragon jus.

TIP

For a lower-carb option, simply replace the Jerusalem artichokes with greens of your choice.

Chicken Kiev, a very flavourful dish of crumbed chicken with a filling of garlic butter and herbs, originated in Russia. Our keto version, using ghee and keto breadcrumbs, is delicious with sweet potato mash. This is wonderful for school or work lunches the next day, so make extra!

CHICKEN KIEV HIGH-CARB DAY

Serves 4

4 chicken breasts (about 300 g each)
190 g (2 cups) keto breadcrumbs (keto bread processed into crumbs)
60 g (½ cup) tapioca flour*
2 eggs
80 ml (⅓ cup) melted coconut oil or good-quality animal fat*
lemon wedges, to serve

Broccoli and garlic butter
3 garlic cloves, finely chopped
100 g Broccoli Rice (page 165), cooked
1 tablespoon finely chopped flat-leaf parsley leaves
¼ teaspoon lemon juice
150 g ghee
sea salt and freshly ground black pepper

* See Glossary

Place all the broccoli and garlic butter ingredients in a bowl and mix well. Season with salt and pepper.

Tear off two 30 cm square sheets of baking paper. Spoon half the broccoli and garlic butter onto one sheet of paper to form a log about 18 cm in length. Repeat this process with the remaining butter and paper. Roll the paper around each butter log, place them on a tray and transfer to the freezer for 20 minutes to firm up.

Meanwhile, using a sharp knife, make a pocket in each chicken breast by cutting along one side. Cut each butter log in half, so you have four equal portions. Fill each pocket with a portion of butter, then tuck the chicken over to enclose the butter filling and secure with a toothpick.

Place the breadcrumbs in a shallow bowl and season with salt and pepper. Mix well and set aside. Place the tapioca flour in another shallow bowl. In a third bowl, whisk the eggs and 3 tablespoons of water until well combined.

Working with one piece at a time, carefully dust the chicken in the tapioca flour, shaking off any excess. Next, dip the chicken in the egg mixture, then evenly and completely coat with the breadcrumbs.

Place the crumbed chicken on a tray and transfer to the fridge to chill for 15 minutes.

Preheat the oven to 180°C (160°C fan-forced).

Heat the coconut oil or animal fat in a large ovenproof frying pan over medium–high heat. Add the chicken and cook on each side for 2 minutes, or until golden. Drain the oil or fat from the pan, transfer to the oven and bake for 15–16 minutes until the chicken is cooked through.

Serve the chicken with the lemon wedges on the side.

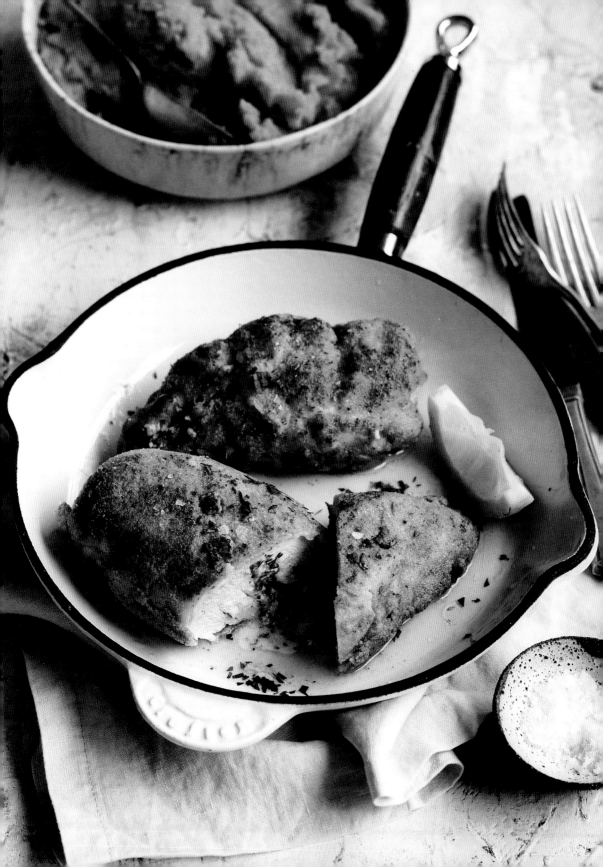

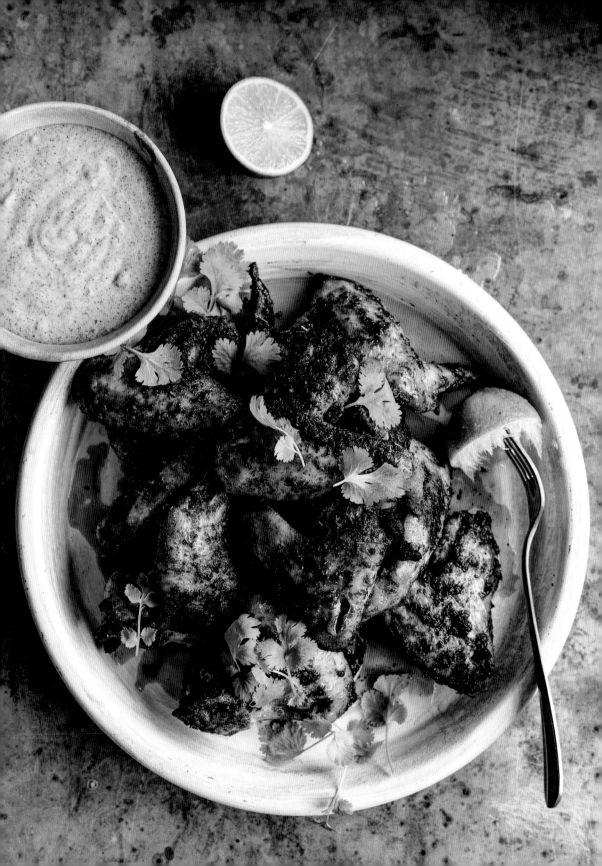

If you have read any of my previous cookbooks, you will know I have a bit of a thing for chicken wings. I think most chefs do, as they are one of the tastiest parts of the chicken and are very affordable and quick to prepare. Because of this, I am always looking for interesting ways in which to serve them. Here, the flavour inspiration is from Peru.

PERUVIAN CHICKEN WINGS WITH AJI VERDE

Serves 4

1.5 kg chicken wings
coriander leaves, to serve
1 lime, halved

Aji verde
2 large handfuls of coriander
   leaves
1 serrano chilli, deseeded
   and chopped
100 g Aioli (page 165)
1 tablespoon olive oil
1 tablespoon apple cider vinegar
sea salt and freshly ground
   black pepper

Spicy marinade
2 tablespoons coconut oil
   or good-quality animal
   fat*, melted
4 garlic cloves, finely chopped
3 tablespoons tamari or
   coconut aminos*
3 tablespoons lime juice
3 tablespoons honey
2 tablespoons chipotle chillies in
   adobo sauce, finely chopped
2 teaspoons ground cumin
2 teaspoons smoked paprika
1 teaspoon finely chopped
   thyme leaves
1 teaspoon sea salt

* See Glossary

For the aji verde, combine the coriander, chilli, aioli, olive oil and vinegar in a blender with a pinch of salt and blend until smooth. Taste and season with salt and pepper. Pour into a small bowl, cover and refrigerate until required.

Combine all the spicy marinade ingredients in a large bowl.

Toss the wings in the spicy marinade and turn to coat well. Cover and marinate in the fridge for 2 hours or, for best results, overnight.

Preheat the oven to 220°C (200°C fan-forced). Line a baking tray with baking paper.

Place the wings in a single layer on the prepared tray and pour over any remaining marinade. Roast, flipping and basting the wings occasionally, for 40 minutes, or until golden and cooked through.

Season the wings with salt and pepper and transfer to a serving platter. Serve scattered with coriander leaves and with the aji verde and lime halves on the side.

Korean spiced roast chicken is something I have wanted to play around with for a while – and this book presented the perfect opportunity. When I tried the result, I was blown away by the way the flavours work so harmoniously together. Team yours with a chilli sauce and some green veg. I hope this recipe becomes a firm family favourite.

KOREAN SPICED ROAST CHICKEN WITH SPICY CUCUMBER SALAD

Serves 4

2 tablespoons lard or other good-quality animal fat*, melted
4 garlic cloves, finely grated
2 tablespoons finely grated ginger
3 tablespoons tamari or coconut aminos*
1 tablespoon fish sauce
3 tablespoons honey
1 x 1.6 kg chicken

Spicy cucumber salad
1 garlic clove, finely grated
2 tablespoons tamari or coconut aminos*
3 tablespoons apple cider vinegar
2 teaspoons Fermented Chilli Sambal (page 172)
1 teaspoon sesame oil
1 teaspoon honey
4 Lebanese cucumbers, halved lengthways and thickly sliced

* See Glossary

Combine the fat, garlic, ginger, tamari or coconut aminos, fish sauce and honey in a large bowl. Add the chicken and rub the marinade over the entire bird. Cover and marinate in the fridge for 2 hours, turning the chicken every 30 minutes to evenly coat with the marinade.

Preheat the oven to 160°C (140°C fan-forced).

Remove the chicken from the bowl (reserve the marinade), place in a roasting tin and allow to stand for 30 minutes to come to room temperature. Pour 300 ml of water around the chicken and roast for 1 hour and 15 minutes, brushing the chicken with the reserved marinade every 10 minutes. Increase the temperature to 180°C (160°C fan-forced) and roast for a further 15 minutes, or until the chicken is golden brown and cooked through. To check, insert a skewer in the thigh; if the juices run clear, the chicken is cooked. Remove from the oven, cover loosely and rest in a warm place for 10 minutes.

Meanwhile, to make the spicy cucumber salad, place the garlic, tamari or coconut aminos, vinegar, chilli sambal, sesame oil and honey in a bowl and mix well. Add the cucumber and gently toss to combine. Stand for 15 minutes to allow the flavours to develop.

Carve the chicken and serve with the spicy cucumber salad.

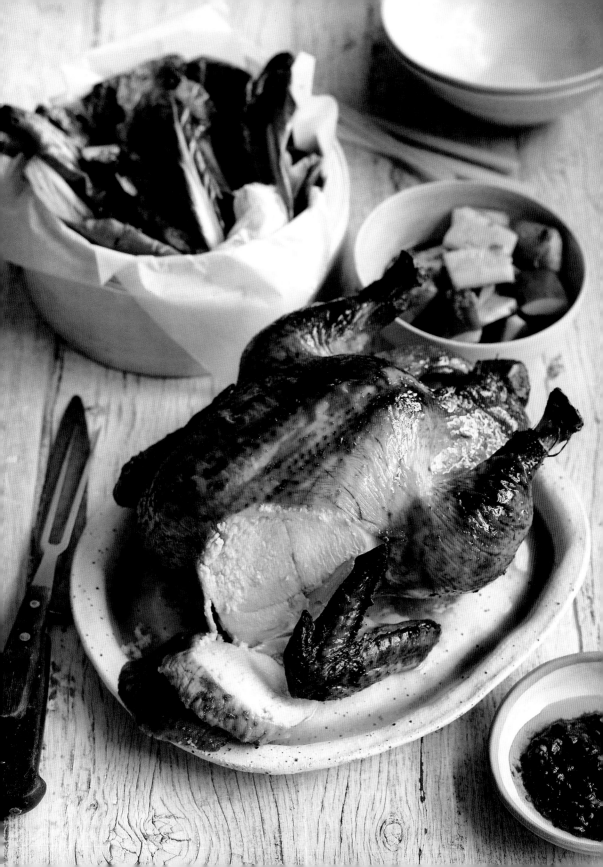

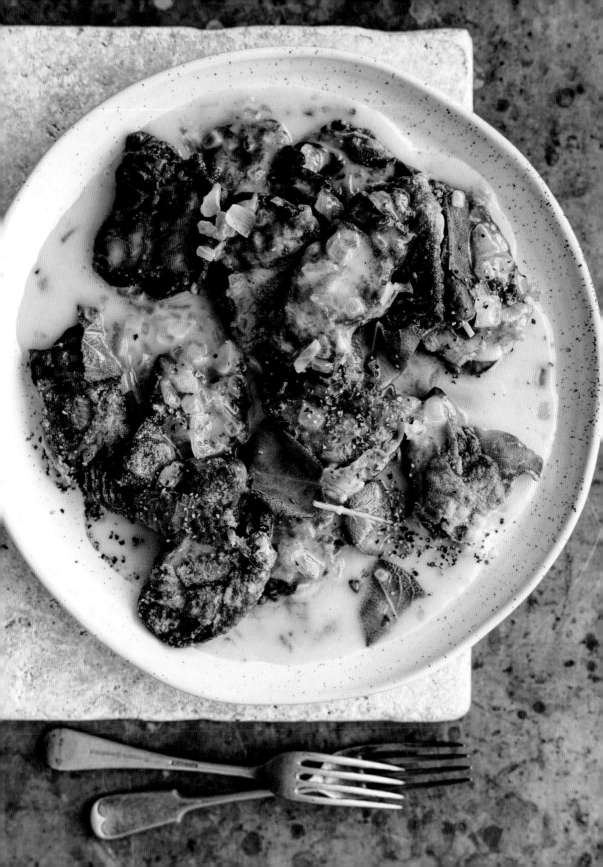

Saltimbocca, which translates as 'jump in the mouth', is a classic Italian dish made with veal wrapped in prosciutto and sage, and cooked in white wine and butter. Here, I have taken the liberty to make my own powerhouse version using chicken livers. And, without sacrificing flavour or texture, I have replaced the butter with ghee or a non-dairy alternative. You could also use duck or veal or chicken thighs, as long as you stay true to the flavourings.

CHICKEN LIVER SALTIMBOCCA

Serves 4

20 chicken livers
sea salt and freshly ground
  black pepper
26 sage leaves
10 thin slices of prosciutto, halved
tapioca flour*, for dusting
200 g ghee or good-quality
  animal fat*
1 onion, chopped
250 ml (1 cup) white wine
  (such as chardonnay)
2 garlic cloves, finely chopped
2 tablespoons coconut cream

* See Glossary

Rinse the chicken livers under cold water and pat dry with paper towel. Trim off any fat, sinew and veins and lightly season with salt and pepper.

Place a sage leaf on each liver, wrap with a piece of prosciutto to enclose and flatten slightly by pressing down with your hands. Lightly dust the wrapped livers with the tapioca flour.

Heat 1 tablespoon of ghee or fat in a large frying pan over medium–high heat, add the wrapped livers in batches and pan-fry for 1 minute on each side until golden. Carefully remove the livers from the pan (the fat may spit) and set aside.

Wipe the pan clean, place over medium heat and add 2 tablespoons of ghee or fat. When the pan is hot, add the onion and sauté for 5 minutes, or until softened. Increase the heat to medium–high, pour in the wine, stir to deglaze and simmer for about 3 minutes until reduced by half. Add the garlic and cook for 1 minute until fragrant.

Reduce the heat to medium, stir in the remaining ghee or fat and the coconut cream, then return the livers to the pan. Cook for 1 minute, carefully flipping the livers halfway through, until they are just cooked and the sauce has thickened to the consistency of pouring cream.

Roughly chop or tear the remaining sage leaves, stir into the sauce and season with salt and pepper. Serve.

Jalfrezi is a very popular curry, in India and throughout the world, because of its tantalising flavour and enticing aroma. I was introduced to this dish by Valerie and Courtney who appeared as a team in an early season of *My Kitchen Rules*. The special curry was from Valerie's beloved father's recipe book he had handed down to his family. You can replace the chicken with duck, pork belly, lamb or beef and, depending on your carb intake, you can serve as is or with some cauliflower and broccoli rice (page 167) or some coconut naan bread (page 171).

CHICKEN JALFREZI

Serves 4–6

6 chicken marylands
sea salt and freshly ground
    black pepper
2 tablespoons coconut oil or
    good-quality animal fat*
1 onion, chopped
6 cardamom pods, crushed
1½ teaspoons cumin seeds
1 tablespoon finely chopped
    ginger
3 garlic cloves, finely chopped
1 green capsicum, deseeded
    and chopped
1 red capsicum, deseeded
    and chopped
1 tablespoon tomato paste
2 teaspoons garam masala
1 teaspoon ground turmeric
1 teaspoon ground coriander
1 teaspoon ground cumin
400 g whole peeled tomatoes,
    crushed (see Note page 66)
250 ml (1 cup) Brown Chicken
    Bone Broth (page 166)
1 pinch of cayenne pepper
1 handful of coriander sprigs

* See Glossary

Preheat the oven to 160°C (140°C fan-forced).

Season the chicken with salt and pepper.

Heat the coconut oil or animal fat in a large flameproof casserole dish over medium–high heat. Add the chicken in batches and brown on each side for 3 minutes, or until golden. Remove from the dish and set aside.

Next, reduce the heat to medium, add the onion to the dish and sauté for 5 minutes, or until softened. Add the cardamom and cumin seeds and cook, stirring, for 1½ minutes, or until the seeds start to pop. Stir in the ginger and garlic and sauté for 30 seconds, or until fragrant. Add the green and red capsicum, tomato paste, garam masala and ground spices and sauté for a further 2 minutes, or until the capsicum is slightly softened. Add the tomatoes, broth and cayenne pepper and season with salt and pepper.

Return the chicken to the dish and bring to a simmer. Cover with the lid, then transfer to the oven to bake for 45–50 minutes, or until the chicken is cooked through.

Scatter the coriander sprigs over the chicken jalfrezi and serve.

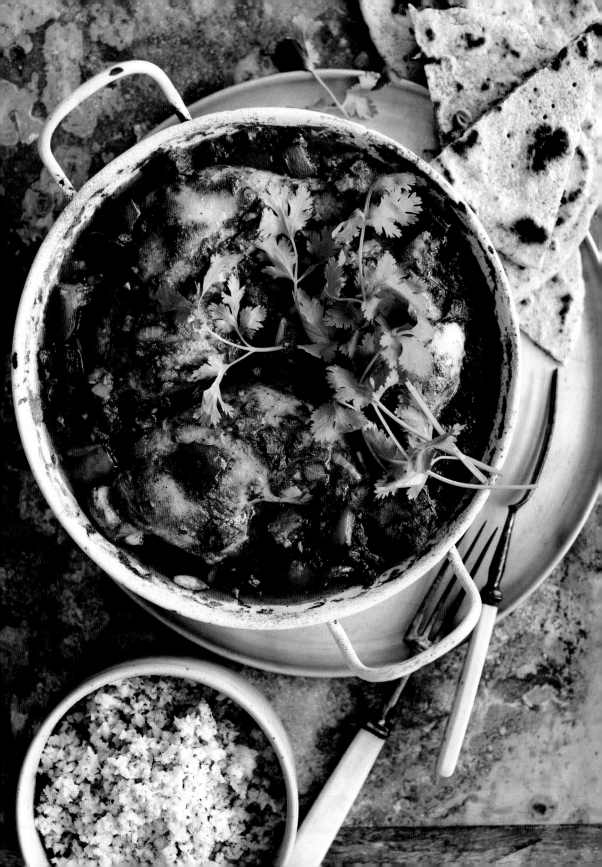

Matzo balls are Jewish soup dumplings usually served in a chicken broth, with or without vegetables. Traditionally, the dumplings are made from unleavened bread; in this healthier keto version, I remove the grains without losing any of the flavour.

CHICKEN MATZO BALL SOUP

Serves 4

2 tablespoons lard or other good-quality animal fat*
2 chicken marylands
1 onion, chopped
3 garlic cloves, finely chopped
2 celery stalks, diced
2 carrots, diced
4 thyme sprigs
2 fresh bay leaves
2 litres Brown Chicken Bone Broth (page 166)
1 handful of tarragon leaves, chopped
1 handful of dill fronds, chopped
1 teaspoon lemon juice
sea salt and freshly ground black pepper

Matzo balls

3 eggs
2 garlic cloves, grated
2 teaspoons finely chopped flat-leaf parsley leaves
¾ teaspoon sea salt
¼ teaspoon freshly ground black pepper
½ teaspoon baking powder
200 g (2 cups) almond meal
2 tablespoons tapioca flour*
2 tablespoons lard or other good-quality animal fat*, melted

* See Glossary

To make the matzo balls, place the eggs, garlic, parsley and salt and pepper in a bowl and whisk to combine. Add the baking powder, almond meal, tapioca flour and fat and mix well. Cover and refrigerate for 1 hour. With clean wet hands, roll the mixture into cherry-sized balls. Return to the fridge until needed.

Melt the fat in a large saucepan over medium–high heat. Add the chicken and cook for 4 minutes on each side to brown. Remove from the pan and set aside.

Reduce the heat to medium. Add the onion to the pan and sauté for 5 minutes, or until softened. Stir in the garlic, celery and carrot and sauté for 5 minutes, or until the vegetables start to colour slightly. Return the chicken to the pan and add the thyme and bay leaves. Pour in the broth, cover with the lid and simmer for 1½ hours, or until the flesh is falling off the bone.

Remove the chicken from the broth and, when cool enough to handle, shred the flesh and discard the bones. Add the shredded chicken to the soup, then add the matzo balls and cover with the lid. Simmer for 10 minutes, or until the matzo balls have expanded and are cooked through. Stir in the tarragon, dill and lemon juice and season with salt and pepper.

Ladle the soup into warm bowls and serve.

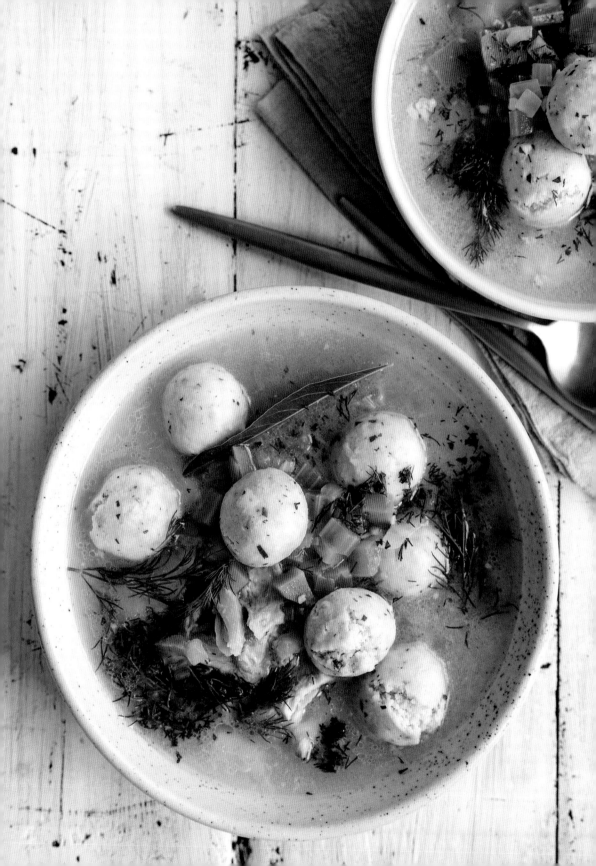

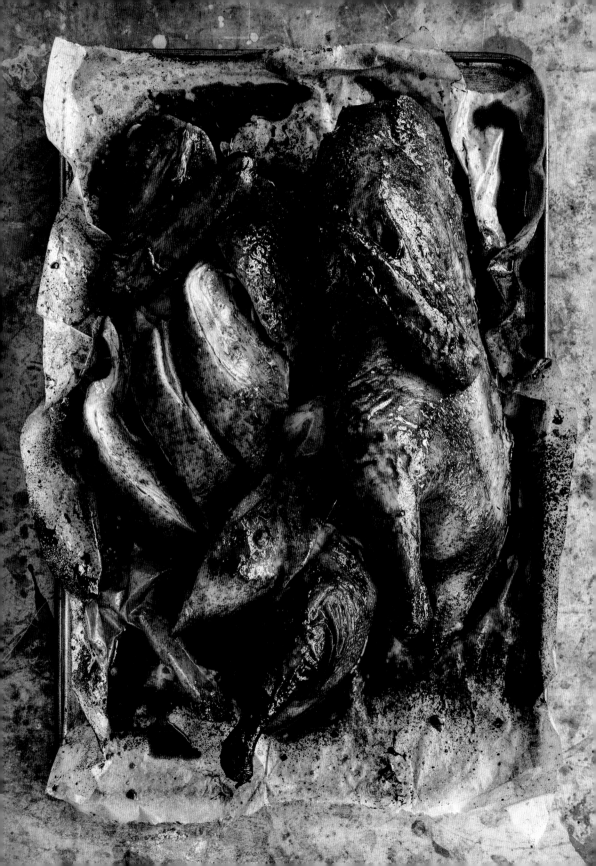

If you have never experienced Peking roast duck, it truly is one of life's greatest culinary experiences. Becoming a Peking duck master takes years and years of training, and there is a big difference between mind-blowing and good. I have to say that the version here, while good, cannot come close to the masters who have studied and perfected their technique over a lifetime. BUT, our home-cooked version definitely results in something delicious and healthy for the whole family to enjoy. I encourage you to give this a try. You'll need to start this recipe one day in advance.

PEKING ROAST DUCK

Serves 4–6

1 x 2 kg duck
1 tablespoon salt
1 tablespoon coconut sugar
2 teaspoons Chinese five spice
3 star anise
200 mls shaoxing wine

Marinade
90 ml apple cider vinegar
80 g honey
150 ml shaoxing wine
2 tablespoons tamari or
    coconut aminos*
½ lemon, halved
1 garlic bulb, halved horizontally
2 cm piece of ginger, sliced
1 spring onion

* See Glossary

Rinse the duck, pat dry with paper towel, then place in a large shallow bowl. Season all over with the salt, sugar and five spice, including in the cavity. Place the star anise in the cavity, then pour the shaoxing wine into the cavity. Weave a metal or bamboo skewer through the overhanging skin along the sides of the cavity to tightly seal and enclose the liquid. Allow to stand for 2 hours in the fridge, uncovered.

Meanwhile, make the marinade. Combine all the ingredients in a saucepan and pour in 250 ml (1 cup) of water. Bring to a simmer, then reduce the heat to low and gently simmer for 30 minutes. Set aside.

When ready, remove the duck from the fridge. Bring the marinade to the boil, then pour over the duck. Pour the marinade from the bottom of the tray back into the pan and bring back to the boil, then pour over the duck again. Remove the duck from the tray, place on a wire rack and transfer to the fridge, uncovered, to allow the skin to dry out overnight. Reserve the marinade.

The next day, preheat the oven to 160°C (140°C fan-forced). Place a wire rack over a roasting tin. Remove the duck from the fridge and allow it to come to room temperature.

Place the duck in the prepared tin and roast for 1 hour 45 minutes, basting with the reserved marinade and flipping over halfway through cooking to ensure the skin cooks evenly. Increase the oven temperature to 180°C (160°C fan-forced) and roast for 20–25 minutes, or until the duck is cooked through and the skin is deep golden and crispy. Cover the skin with baking paper if it starts to darken too much during cooking. Allow to rest for 20 minutes, keeping warm.

Carve the duck and serve.

There is chicken and then there is SOUTHERN FRIED CHICKEN from the US of A! Never has chicken tasted better: there is something just so pleasurable about biting through a crispy outer crust to find juicy melt-in-the-mouth chicken and a combination of spices that dance on your tastebuds. I encourage you to give this a go one weekend and get the whole family involved in the process so it becomes a team event.

SOUTHERN FRIED CHICKEN

Serves 4–6

4 eggs
2 tablespoons almond milk
150 g hemp or tapioca flour*, for coating
1 x 1.8 kg chicken, cut into 10 pieces
coconut oil or good-quality animal fat*, for deep-frying
200 g Aioli (page 165)
80 ml (⅓ cup) Hot Sauce (page 174)
sea salt
lemon wedges, to serve

Spice mix

3 tablespoons psyllium husks*
30 g (¼ cup) tapioca flour*
200 g (2 cups) almond meal
2 teaspoons dried oregano
2 teaspoons dried basil
½ teaspoon chilli powder
2 teaspoons freshly ground black pepper
2 teaspoons sea salt
1 teaspoon sweet paprika
2 teaspoons ground cumin
2 teaspoons garlic powder
2 teaspoons onion powder

* See Glossary

Preheat the oven to 180°C (160°C fan-forced).

Place all the spice mix ingredients in a shallow bowl and mix well.

Whisk the eggs and almond milk in another shallow bowl. Place the hemp or tapioca flour in a third bowl.

One at a time, toss the chicken pieces in the flour and dust off the excess. Then dip in the egg mixture, followed by the spice mixture, turning and pressing gently to coat thoroughly.

Add enough coconut oil or animal fat to fill a large saucepan by one-third and heat to 160°C over medium–high heat. (To test, drop a small piece of chicken into the oil – it should bubble instantly around the edges.) Add the chicken in batches and fry for 3–4 minutes until golden. Remove with a slotted spoon and drain on paper towel. Transfer the chicken to a baking tray and roast for 10–15 minutes until cooked through.

Spoon the aioli into a small serving bowl, then swirl through the hot sauce.

Season the chicken with salt and serve with the aioli dipping sauce and the lemon wedges on the side.

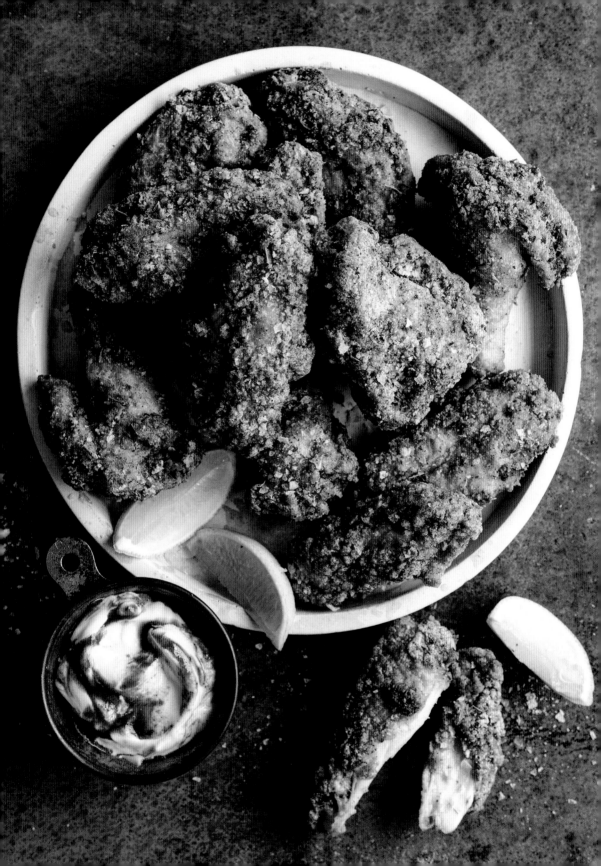

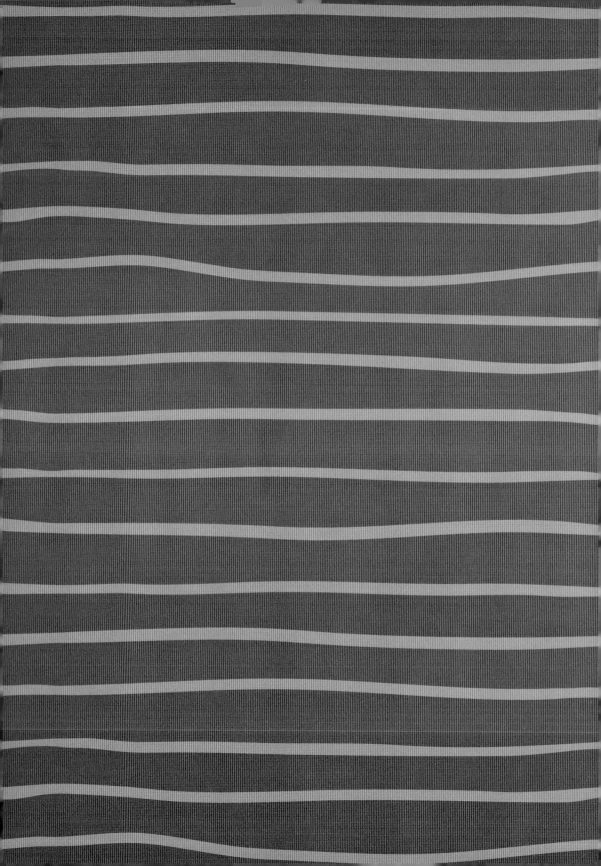

PORK

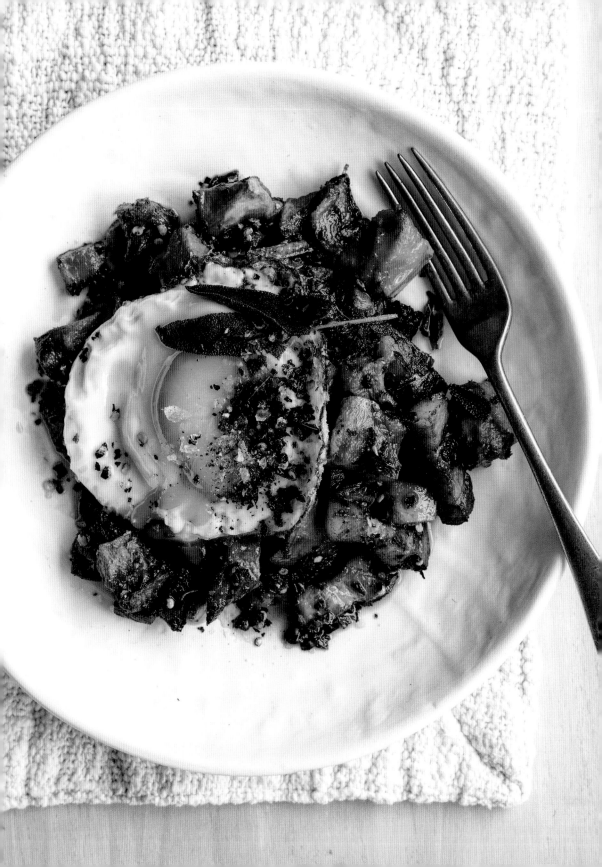

Good ol' bacon and eggs have been given a little makeover here by adding two ingredients that go so well together: pumpkin and sage. Their addition elevates this dish to brand new heights and makes for a very yummy breakfast, lunch or dinner.

FRIED EGGS WITH SAGE, PUMPKIN AND SPECK

Serves 4

500 g kent pumpkin, cut into
   2 cm dice
200 g speck, diced
80 ml (⅓ cup) melted coconut oil
   or good-quality animal fat*
sea salt and freshly ground
   black pepper
1 handful of sage leaves, torn
4 eggs

* See Glossary

Preheat the oven to 220°C (200°C fan-forced).

Place the pumpkin and speck on a baking tray, drizzle over 2 tablespoons of the coconut oil or animal fat, toss to coat and spread out in a single layer. Season with salt and pepper. Roast for 20 minutes, or until the pumpkin is almost cooked through. Scatter over half the sage leaves, gently toss and continue to roast for 10 minutes, or until the pumpkin is golden and tender.

Meanwhile, heat 1 tablespoon of the oil or fat in a large non-stick frying pan over medium heat. Crack in the eggs and fry for 2–2½ minutes until the egg whites are set (or cook to your liking). Season with salt and pepper, remove from the pan and set aside.

Heat the remaining oil or fat in the same pan over medium–high heat. Add the remaining sage leaves and fry for 15 seconds, or until just starting to colour. Remove the sage from the pan and place on paper towel to drain. Season with a pinch of salt.

Divide the pumpkin and speck between serving plates, top with a fried egg and scatter over the fried sage. Finish with a good grind of pepper to serve.

A huge platter of meatballs is every family's saviour when it comes to a quick, budget-friendly and extremely delicious weeknight dinner. These Vietnamese-inspired pork meatballs will have everyone wishing they were on the table every week. All you need are some lettuce cups to wrap them up in.

VIETNAMESE PORK MEATBALLS

Serves 4

coconut oil or good-quality
  animal fat*, for greasing
3 garlic cloves, finely chopped
1 lemongrass stem, pale part
  only, finely chopped
1 French shallot, finely chopped
1 teaspoon finely grated ginger
3 teaspoons fish sauce
1 tablespoon chopped
  coriander leaves
2 bird's eye chillis, deseeded and
  finely chopped (optional)
3 tablespoons coconut cream
500 g pork mince
1 large handful of mixed Asian
  herbs (such as Vietnamese mint
  and coriander)

Nuoc cham
3 tablespoons apple
  cider vinegar
3 tablespoons honey
3 tablespoons fish sauce
2 small red chillies, deseeded
  and finely chopped
1 garlic clove, finely grated
juice of 2 limes
2 teaspoons finely chopped
  coriander roots and stalks

* See Glossary

To make the nuoc cham, place the vinegar, honey, fish sauce, chilli and garlic in a small saucepan and stir to combine. Bring to a simmer over medium heat, reduce the heat to low and simmer, stirring occasionally, for 5 minutes to allow the flavours to develop. Mix in the lime juice and coriander and set aside to cool.

Meanwhile, preheat the oven to 200°C (180°C fan-forced). Lightly grease a baking tray with the coconut oil or animal fat.

Place the garlic, lemongrass, shallot, ginger, fish sauce, coriander, chilli (if using) and coconut cream in a food processor and pulse a few times. Scrape down the side of the bowl, add the pork mince and process for 10 seconds to combine.

Roll the pork mixture into walnut-sized balls and place on the prepared tray in a single layer. Bake for 8–10 minutes until the meatballs are cooked through.

Arrange the meatballs and herbs on a platter. Drizzle over some nuoc cham and serve with the rest of the nuoc cham on the side.

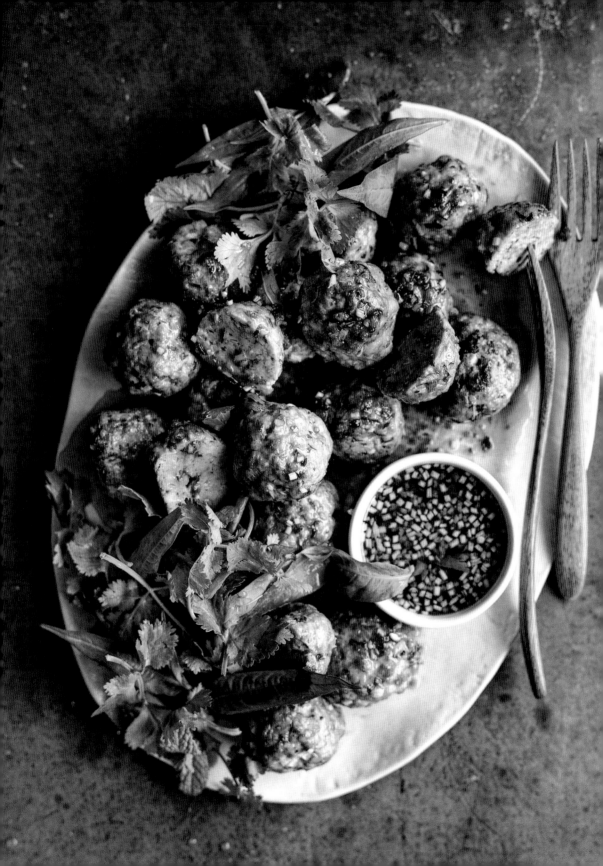

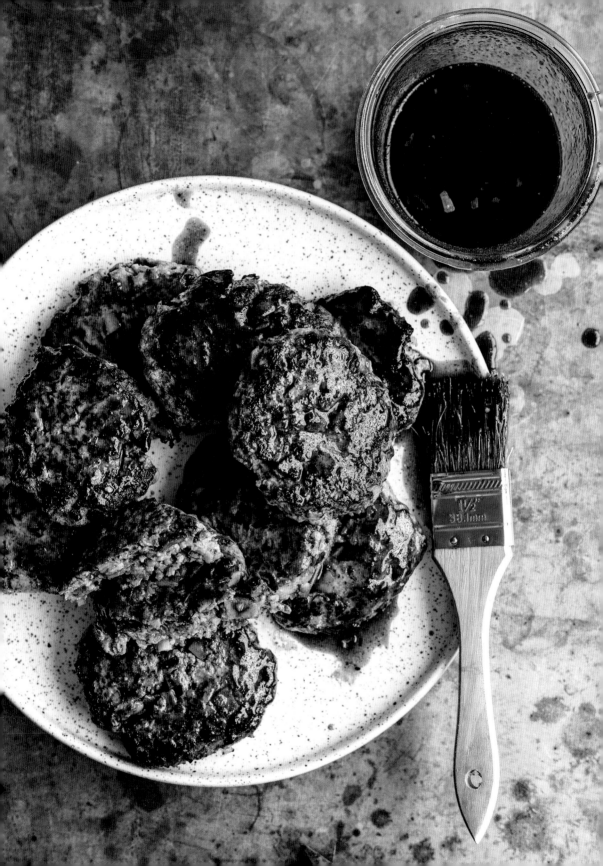

If you are going to have a burger, then why not go the whole hog – literally – and create these amazing patties that combine pork mince with the yumminess of bacon? To go all in, blood sausage would make for a great addition, too. The key with patties is to season them well so they aren't bland. Once they are grilled, you can construct the burger of your dreams and go naked (no bun) or add your favourite keto bun. Don't forget to include your favourite salad ingredients and sauce.

GLAZED PORK AND BACON BURGERS

Serves 4–6

4 rindless bacon rashers, finely chopped
3 tablespoons coconut oil or good-quality animal fat*
1 onion, finely chopped
150 g mushrooms, finely chopped
2 garlic cloves, finely chopped
2 teaspoons finely chopped thyme leaves
1 tablespoon finely chopped flat-leaf parsley leaves
550 g pork mince
1 egg
1 teaspoon sea salt
1 teaspoon freshly ground black pepper
150 ml Smoky Barbecue Sauce (page 178)

* See Glossary

Heat a large frying pan over medium–high heat. Add the bacon and sauté for 5 minutes, or until lightly golden. Transfer the bacon to a bowl and set aside.

Wipe the pan clean, then heat 1 tablespoon of the coconut oil or animal fat over medium heat. Add the onion and sauté for 5 minutes until softened. Next, add the mushroom and garlic and cook for 3 minutes until softened. Transfer the onion and mushroom mixture to the bacon and allow to cool completely.

Add the thyme, parsley, pork mince, egg, salt and pepper to the cooled bacon mixture, then mix well to combine. Shape the mixture into ten patties.

Heat a large frying pan over medium–high heat. Add the remaining oil or fat and cook the patties in batches for 3 minutes on each side, or until cooked through. Transfer to a plate and allow to rest for 2 minutes. Whisk any juices in the pan into the smoky barbecue sauce.

Brush the smoky barbecue sauce over the patties to glaze, then serve.

*If you have never tried pork belly, I highly recommend you give it a go.
You can eat this dish either hot or cold, and the dressing works on it either way.
Steamed bok choy with sesame oil and sesame seeds and a side of kimchi
are all you need if you feel like adding some greens.*

PORK BELLY WITH SICHUAN AND CHILLI DRESSING

Serves 4

800 g boned pork belly, skin
  scored, at room temperature
4 cm piece of ginger, finely sliced
2 spring onions, roughly chopped
1 teaspoon Sichuan peppercorns
sea salt
2 tablespoons Typhoon Garlic
  (page 179)

Sichuan and chilli dressing
2 teaspoons Sichuan peppercorns
1 teaspoon finely grated ginger
1 spring onion, white part
  finely chopped, green part
  finely sliced
½ teaspoon sea salt
200 ml Chilli Oil (page 169)
1½ tablespoons tamari or
  coconut aminos*
2 tablespoons apple cider vinegar

Place the pork belly in a large saucepan and fill with cold water. Add the ginger, spring onion, Sichuan peppercorns and a good pinch of salt. Bring to the boil over medium–high heat, then reduce the heat to low and gently simmer for 1 hour, or until the pork is tender and cooked through. Remove the pork from the liquid and set aside, keeping warm. Bring the liquid back to the boil.

To make the Sichuan and chilli dressing, place the Sichuan peppercorns in a frying pan over medium heat and cook, tossing frequently, for 30–40 seconds until fragrant and toasted. Allow to cool, then coarsely grind using a spice grinder or mortar and pestle. Next, combine the ginger, spring onion whites, salt and toasted Sichuan pepper in a small bowl. Pour in 3 tablespoons of the boiling pork-cooking water, mix well, and allow to infuse for 10 minutes, or until cool. To finish, mix in the chilli oil, tamari or coconut aminos and vinegar.

Cut the pork belly into thick slices and arrange on a platter. Season with some salt, sprinkle over the typhoon garlic, then pour over the Sichuan and chilli dressing. Sprinkle with the spring onion greens and serve.

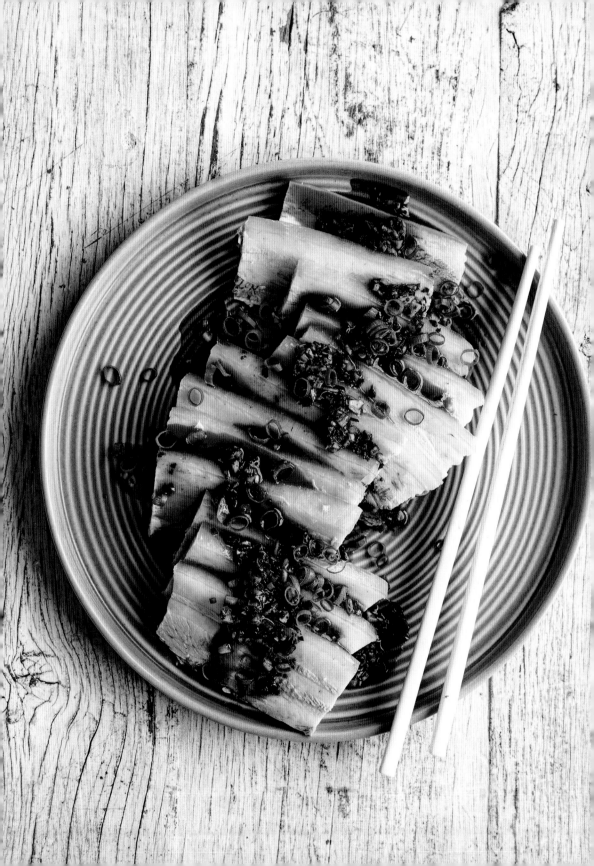

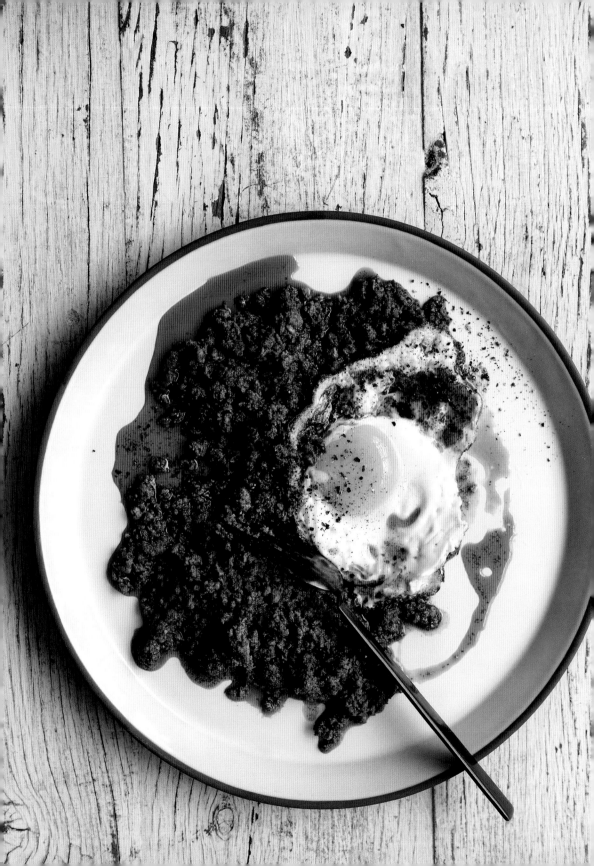

Did you know there are two types of chorizo: the Spanish/Portuguese sausage and a heavily spiced and flavoured Mexican mince meat? I love both styles, but for speed and ease, I find mince is the way to go as I always have some in the freezer, along with the spices on hand to create this meal. Serve with fried or poached eggs and you have a perfect breakfast, lunch or dinner. If you like, add some greens like spinach or sprouts.

MEXICAN CHORIZO MINCE WITH FRIED EGGS

Serves 4

2 tablespoons coconut oil or
good-quality animal fat*
sea salt and freshly ground
black pepper
4 eggs

Mexican chorizo mince
600 g coarse pork mince
(ask your butcher)
200 g pork fat, coarsely minced
(ask your butcher)
6 garlic cloves, finely chopped
1 teaspoon chilli powder
2½ tablespoons sweet paprika
2 teaspoons smoked paprika
1½ teaspoons sea salt
1 tablespoon dried oregano
½ teaspoon freshly ground
black pepper
1 teaspoon ground cumin
1 teaspoon ground coriander
¼ teaspoon ground cloves
80 ml (⅓ cup) apple cider
vinegar

* See Glossary

Place all the Mexican chorizo mince ingredients in a bowl and mix well to combine. Cover and marinate in the fridge for 2 hours or, for best results, overnight.

When you're ready to cook, heat 1 tablespoon of the coconut oil or animal fat in a large frying pan over medium–high heat. Add the chorizo mince and, stirring with a wooden spoon to break up the lumps, cook for 5 minutes, or until browned. Pour in 250 ml (1 cup) of water and bring to the boil. Turn down the heat to medium and simmer for 10 minutes, or until the liquid has reduced. Season with a little salt and pepper if needed.

Meanwhile, heat the remaining oil or fat in a large non-stick frying pan over medium heat. Crack in the eggs and fry for 2–2½ minutes until the egg whites are set (or cook to your liking). Season with salt and pepper.

Spoon the chorizo mince onto serving plates, then top with a fried egg and serve.

Crispy pork belly crackling has to be one of life's greatest pleasures. I know in my family we all love the crackling, and if I'm not careful, one of my daughters will pinch mine from my plate when I'm not looking. The combination of crispy pork with the low-carb salad ingredients featured here will keep you in ketosis; and the lovely balance of salty, fatty, meaty and fresh flavours are tied together with an absolutely stellar dressing.

THAI PORK SALAD

Serves 4

1 kg boned pork belly, skin scored, at room temperature
250 ml (1 cup) boiling water
1 tablespoon lard
sea salt
200 g Chinese cabbage (wombok), finely shredded
1 Lebanese cucumber, halved lengthways, deseeded and cut into matchsticks
½ green papaya, cut into matchsticks
2 spring onions, cut into matchsticks
2 French shallots, finely sliced
1 bird's eye chilli, finely sliced
1 large handful of mint leaves
1 large handful of Thai basil leaves
1 large handful of coriander leaves
1 large handful of Vietnamese mint leaves
1 pinch of chilli powder (optional)
lime cheeks, to serve

Dressing

2 bird's eye chillies, deseeded and finely chopped
3 teaspoons finely grated ginger
3 garlic cloves, finely chopped
2 tablespoons coconut sugar
100 ml lime juice
3 tablespoons fish sauce

Place all the dressing ingredients in a high-speed blender and blend until smooth.

Preheat the oven to 240°C (220°C fan-forced) – you need to start by blasting the pork with heat.

Place the pork belly on a wire rack in the kitchen sink, carefully pour the boiling water all over the skin, then pat dry with paper towel.

Rub the pork skin with the lard and season with a good amount of salt. Place the pork in a large roasting tin and roast for 35–40 minutes until the skin starts to bubble. Reduce the temperature to 150°C (130°C fan-forced) and continue to roast the pork for 1 hour 15 minutes, or until the flesh is very tender. Transfer to a plate and allow to rest for 15 minutes, keeping warm. If the crackling isn't crisp enough, place the pork, crackling-side up, under a hot grill for a few minutes.

Cut the pork into bite-sized pieces and set aside.

Arrange the cabbage, cucumber, green papaya, spring onion and shallot on a large platter. Scatter over the pork and chilli, then drizzle over the dressing. Sprinkle on the herbs and chilli powder (if using) and serve with the lime cheeks for a bit of extra zing.

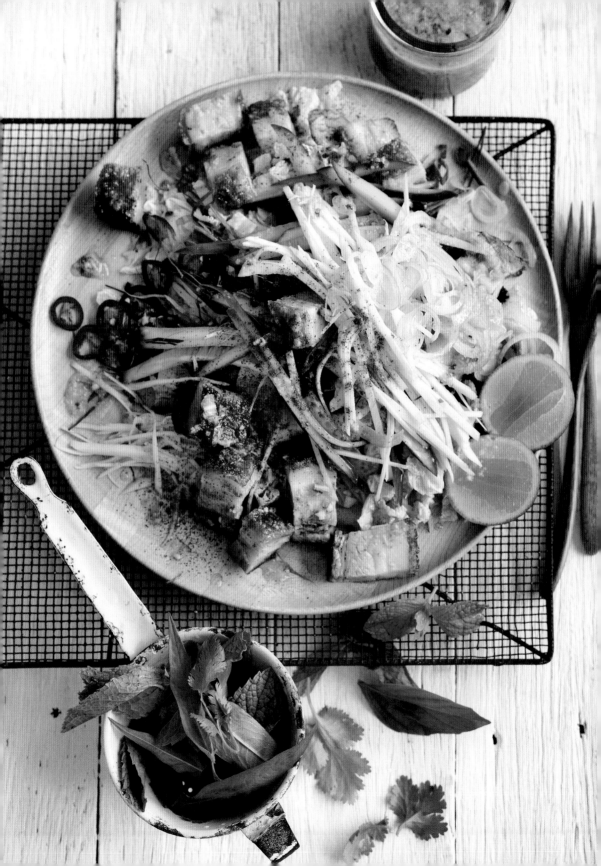

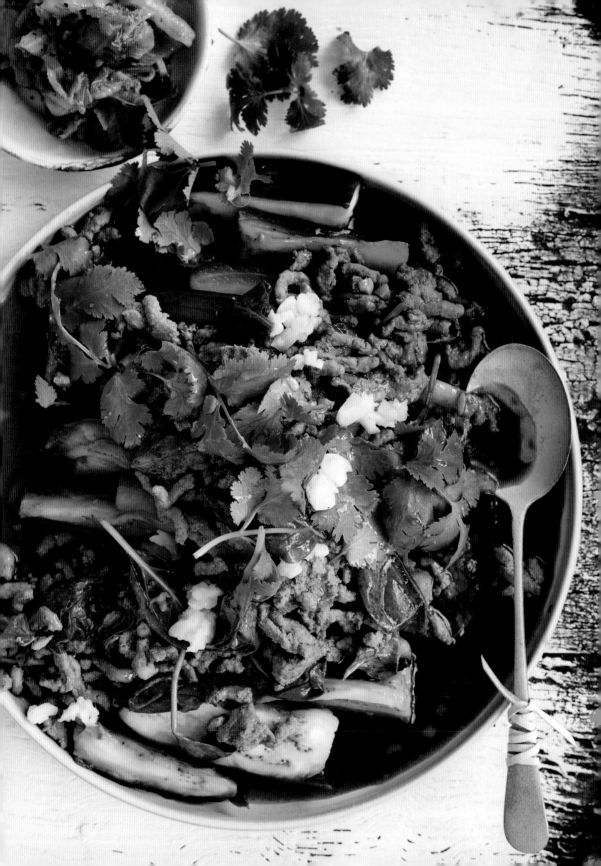

Anything made with pork mince is a winner, but when it comes to Chinese-flavoured pork mince, we are talking a whole other level. This classic dish is a wonderful combination of eggplant, pork and garlic. The key when working with eggplant is to cook it all the way through so it becomes super tender.

SPICED EGGPLANT AND PORK MINCE `HIGH-CARB DAY`

Serves 4

600 g pork mince
3 tablespoons shaoxing wine
1 tablespoon tamari or
  coconut aminos*
3 tablespoons coconut oil or
  good-quality animal fat*
3 garlic cloves, finely chopped
1 tablespoon finely chopped
  ginger
6 Chinese eggplants, halved
  lengthways, then quartered
125 ml (½ cup) Brown Chicken
  Bone Broth (page 166)
3 handfuls of baby spinach leaves
1 teaspoon sesame oil
1 handful of coriander leaves
kimchi, to serve
6–8 Quick Pickled Garlic cloves
  (page 176), crushed

Sauce
2 teaspoons tapioca flour*, mixed
  with 2 tablespoons water
125 ml (½ cup) Brown Chicken
  Bone Broth (page 166)
2 tablespoons Fermented Chilli
  Sambal (page 172)
1 teaspoon honey
2 teaspoons fish sauce
1 tablespoon pickling liquid from
  Quick Pickled Garlic (page 176)
1½ teaspoons tamari or
  coconut aminos*

* See Glossary

Place the pork mince in a bowl, add the shaoxing wine and tamari or coconut aminos and set aside to marinate.

Heat 2 tablespoons of the coconut oil or animal fat in a large saucepan over medium heat, add half the garlic and ginger and sauté for 1 minute, or until fragrant. Add the eggplant and broth and cover with the lid. Cook for 3 minutes, or until the eggplant is half cooked through.

Meanwhile, heat the remaining oil or fat in a large frying pan over medium heat. Add the remaining garlic and ginger and cook for 1 minute, or until fragrant. Add the pork mince mixture and cook, stirring with a wooden spoon to break up the lumps, for 10 minutes, or until browned.

Combine the sauce ingredients in a bowl and mix well.

Stir the sauce into the pork and bring to the boil. Reduce the heat to low and simmer for 5 minutes, or until the sauce thickens.

Pour the mince and sauce over the eggplant, cover and simmer over medium–low heat for 5 minutes. Gently stir in the spinach, cover and cook for a further 5 minutes, or until the eggplant is cooked through. Drizzle over the sesame oil.

Scatter the coriander leaves over the mince and, for a little more spice and probiotic goodness, serve with kimchi and pickled garlic on the side.

The simple pleasure of braising a deliciously fatty piece of pork to the point where it is falling apart is what cooking is all about. And when it is spiced and flavoured so it is mouth-wateringly yummy, all you need to finish it off are some lettuce cups, guacamole, fresh coriander and pickled onion.

PULLED PORK LETTUCE TACOS

Serves 6

1.8 kg boneless pork shoulder, skin and half the fat removed (save the fat for rendering, see page 176, and the skin for crackling), at room temperature
sea salt and freshly ground black pepper
3 fresh bay leaves
400 ml Beef or Brown Chicken Bone Broth (page 165 or 166)

Paste
6 garlic cloves, peeled
1 tablespoon coriander roots, roughly chopped
1 onion, roughly chopped
1 jalapeno chilli, deseeded
3 tablespoons apple cider vinegar
3 tablespoons lard or other good-quality animal fat*
2 tablespoons chipotle chillies in adobo sauce
3 tablespoons tomato paste
1 tablespoon smoked paprika
1 tablespoon ground cumin

Guacamole
3 avocados, mashed with a fork
1 teaspoon ground coriander
1 teaspoon ground cumin
juice of 1–2 limes
1 tablespoon olive oil

To serve
baby cos lettuce leaves
Pickled Red Onion (page 174)
shredded cabbage leaves
coriander sprigs
lime cheeks

* See Glossary

Place all the paste ingredients in a food processor and blitz until a wet but slightly chunky paste forms.

Season the pork with salt and pepper and place in a large casserole dish. Spread the paste over the pork and press the bay leaves on top. Cover and marinate in the fridge for 2 hours or, for best results, overnight.

When you're ready to cook, preheat the oven to 140°C (120°C fan-forced).

Pour the beef or chicken broth around the pork into the dish, cover with the lid and braise for 4 hours, or until the pork is tender. Remove the pork from the liquid and set aside, keeping warm. Place the casserole dish with the liquid over medium–high heat and cook for about 10 minutes, stirring occasionally, until the liquid has reduced by half. Meanwhile, shred the pork. When the liquid has reduced by half, add the shredded pork back to the casserole dish and stir for 3 minutes to heat through. Season with a little more salt and pepper if needed.

Place all the guacamole ingredients in a bowl, season with salt to taste and mix to combine.

Spoon the pulled pork into serving bowls and serve with lettuce leaves, pickled red onion, cabbage, coriander sprigs, guacamole and lime cheeks.

TIP

Any leftover pulled pork can be stored in the freezer for up to 3 months.

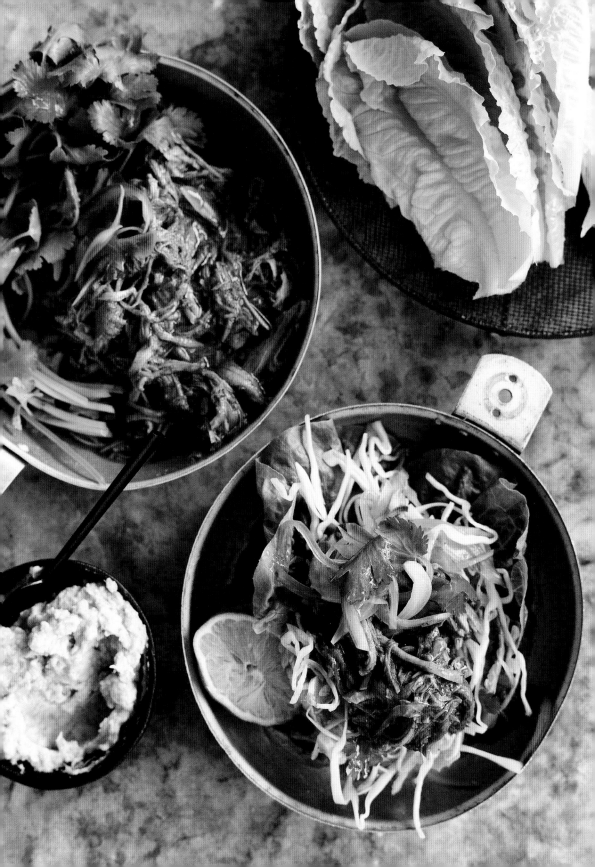

The Filipino dish adobo is super simple and super yummy and can be made with pretty much any meat you like. My favourite is the ever-delicious pork belly. For a wicked weekend dinner, serve with some greens or salad on the side and your choice of fermented veg.

PORK BELLY ADOBO

Serves 4

125 ml (½ cup) tamari or
  coconut aminos*
2 tablespoons honey
1 tablespoon black peppercorns
1.3 kg boned pork belly, cut into
  2 cm thick slices
2 tablespoons coconut oil or
  good-quality animal fat*
1 onion, chopped
10 garlic cloves, halved
  lengthways
5 fresh bay leaves
375 ml (1½ cups) apple
  cider vinegar
sea salt

* See Glossary

Combine the tamari or coconut aminos, honey and peppercorns in a large bowl. Add the pork and toss well to evenly coat. Cover and marinate in the fridge for 2 hours or, for best results, overnight.

When you're ready to cook, preheat the oven to 140°C (120°C fan-forced).

Remove the pork, shake off the excess marinade and place on a plate. Reserve the marinade for braising the pork.

Heat the coconut oil or animal fat in a large flameproof casserole dish over medium–high heat. Add the pork in batches and sear for 2 minutes on each side, or until browned. Transfer to a chopping board, cut into 3 cm pieces and set aside.

Reduce the heat to medium, add the onion to the dish and sauté for 5 minutes, or until softened. Add the garlic and cook for a further 1 minute, or until it starts to colour.

Return the pork to the dish. Add the reserved marinade, the bay leaves, vinegar and 250 ml (1 cup) of water and bring to the boil. Season with a little salt, cover with the lid and braise in the oven for 3–3½ hours, or until the meat is tender.

Divide the pork belly adobo between serving bowls and serve.

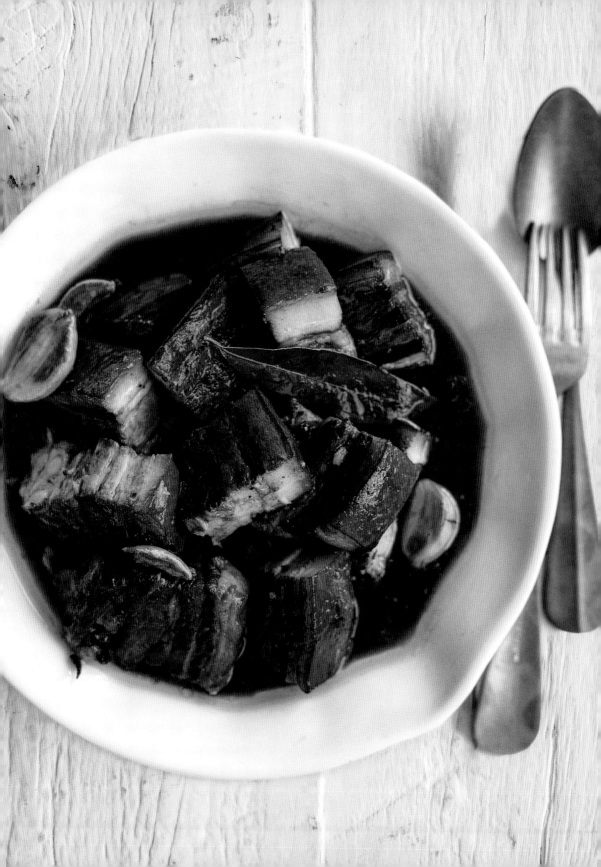

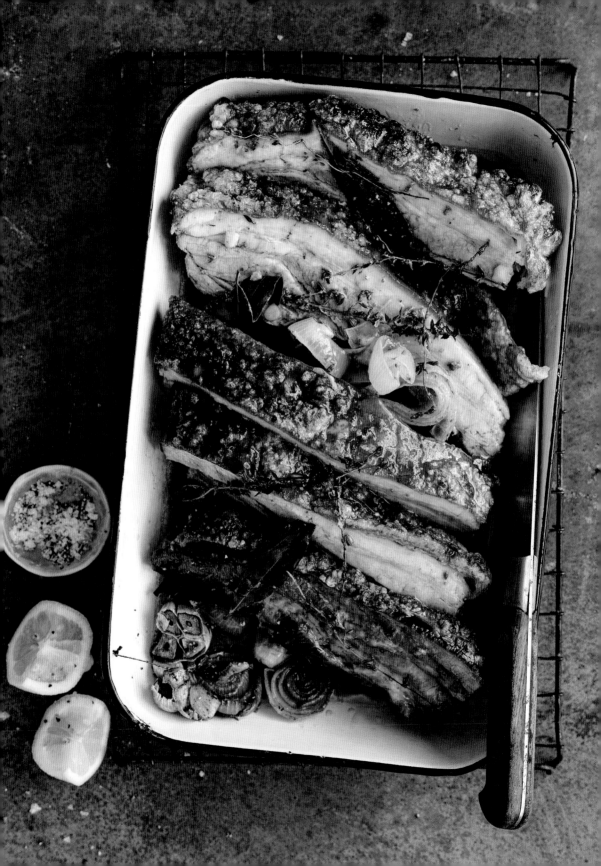

The classic roast pork belly never fails to impress the whole family, and when it comes to leftovers, it's truly the gift that keeps on giving. Together, fennel and pork work a treat and for this reason I wanted to keep this recipe as simple as possible. All you need to add is some apple sauce, mustard or hot sauce (page 174), plus your veg or salad of choice.

ROAST PORK BELLY WITH FENNEL

Serves 4

1.2 kg boned pork belly, skin scored, at room temperature
250 ml (1 cup) boiling water
2 tablespoons coconut oil or good-quality animal fat*, melted
sea salt and freshly ground black pepper
1 tablespoon fennel seeds, toasted and coarsely ground
2 onions, sliced into rounds
1 large fennel bulb, thickly sliced
1 head of garlic, halved horizontally
15 thyme sprigs
2 fresh bay leaves
350 ml Brown Chicken Bone Broth (page 166)
1 teaspoon Dijon mustard
lemon wedges, to serve

* See Glossary

Preheat the oven to 240°C (220°C fan-forced) – you need to start by blasting the pork with heat.

Place the pork belly on a wire rack in the kitchen sink, carefully pour the boiling water all over the skin, then pat dry with paper towel.

Rub the pork skin with the coconut oil or animal fat and season with a good amount of salt. Rub the ground fennel into the flesh and place the pork in a large roasting tin. Roast for 30 minutes, or until the skin starts to bubble. Remove the tin from the oven, carefully lift out the pork and place on a plate.

Reduce the oven temperature to 140°C (120°C fan-forced).

Scatter the onion, fennel slices, garlic, thyme and bay leaves into the tin. Pour in the broth, mix in the mustard and season with salt and pepper. Return the pork to the tin and continue to roast for 1 hour 15 minutes, or until the flesh is very tender. Transfer the pork to a plate and rest for 15 minutes, keeping warm. If the crackling isn't crisp enough, place the pork, crackling-side up, under a hot grill for a few minutes.

Increase the oven temperature to 200°C (180°C fan-forced). Return the tin to the oven and roast the veggies for 10 minutes, or until golden.

Carve the pork belly into thick slices and serve with the roasted veggies and the lemon wedges on the side.

BEEF

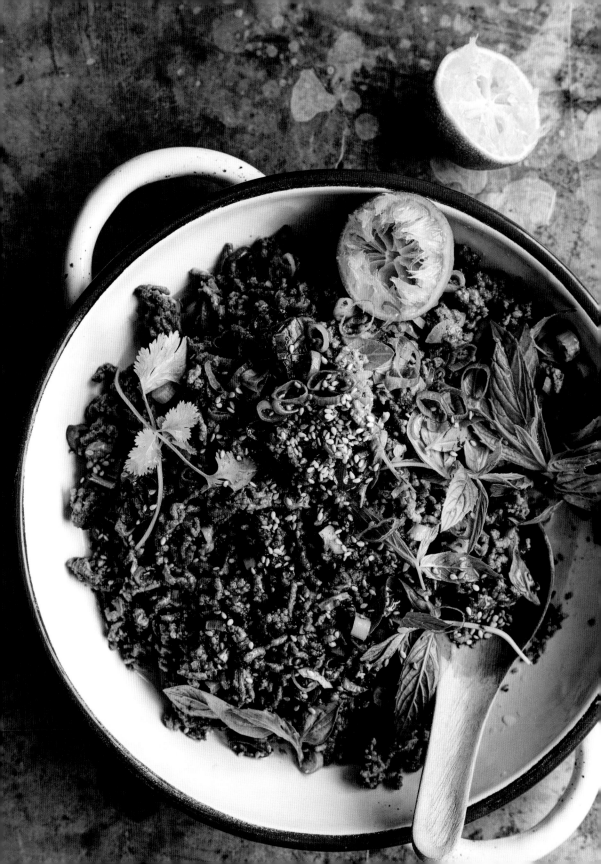

Although larb (or larp) has its origins in Laos, it is one of the main dishes you come across when travelling from village to village in neighbouring Thailand. This traditional salad consists of mince meat or seafood, eaten raw or cooked, with a killer dressing of lime juice, fish sauce, chilli and fresh herbs. Usually served with roasted crushed rice, I have taken the liberty of substituting the rice with sesame seeds. Delicious!

BEEF LARB

Serves 4–6

1 tablespoon sesame seeds
2 tablespoons coconut oil or good-quality animal fat*
600 g beef mince
80 ml (⅓ cup) lime juice
2 tablespoons fish sauce, plus extra if needed
½–1 bird's eye chilli, finely sliced (depending on how spicy you like it)
4 red Asian shallots, finely diced
4 spring onions, green part only, finely sliced, plus extra to serve
1 handful of mint leaves
1 handful of coriander leaves
1 small handful of Thai basil leaves

* See Glossary

Place a wok or frying pan over medium–high heat, add the sesame seeds and cook, tossing constantly, for 1–2 minutes until the sesame seeds are golden and toasted. Remove from the pan and set aside to cool.

Wipe the pan clean, place over medium–high heat and heat the coconut oil or animal fat. Add the mince and cook, stirring with a wooden spoon to break up the lumps, for 6 minutes, or until browned and crumbly. Stir in the lime juice, fish sauce, chilli, shallot and spring onion. Remove from the heat and leave to cool for 1 minute.

Toss half the mint, coriander, Thai basil and sesame seeds through the beef mince. Taste and add a little more fish sauce if needed. Sprinkle over the remaining sesame seeds for a nice crunchy texture and serve with the remaining herbs.

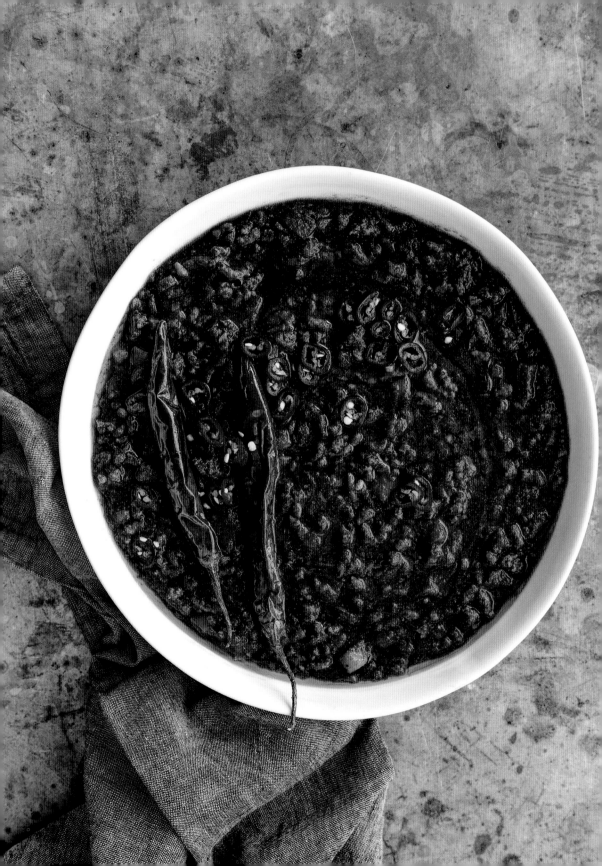

Chilli con carne translates to 'chilli with meat', and that is exactly the type of recipe I love to cook. Like a Mexican version of an Italian bolognese, it can be used in so many ways, from filling keto tacos and tortillas to topping sweet potato nachos or fries and making cottage pies. Or you can simply enjoy a big bowl by itself with some salad on the side.

CHILLI CON CARNE

Serves 4–6

2 tablespoons coconut oil or good-quality animal fat*
1 onion, finely chopped
1 large carrot, chopped
½ red capsicum, deseeded and chopped
3 garlic cloves, finely chopped
1–2 long red chillies, deseeded and finely chopped
600 g beef mince
2 teaspoons smoked paprika
2 teaspoons ground cumin
1 teaspoon ground coriander
¼ teaspoon chilli powder (add another ¼ teaspoon if you like it extra spicy)
2½ teaspoons dried oregano
2½ tablespoons tomato paste
400 g diced tomatoes (see Note page 66)
250 ml (1 cup) Beef Bone Broth (page 165), plus extra if needed
sea salt and freshly ground black pepper

* See Glossary

Heat the coconut oil or animal fat in a large frying pan over medium heat. Add the onion, carrot and capsicum and cook for 8 minutes, or until softened. Stir in the garlic and chilli and cook for 1 minute, or until fragrant.

Add the beef mince to the pan and cook, stirring with a wooden spoon to break up the lumps, for 5 minutes, or until browned. Add the spices, oregano and tomato paste and cook for 1 minute, then mix in the tomatoes and broth. Reduce the heat to low and simmer for 30 minutes, adding more broth if needed. Season with salt and a good grind of pepper and serve.

One of my all-time favourite childhood memories is eating a pie for breakfast before school. Not much has changed, except I now make my own pies.

CURRIED BEEF PIES WITH PARSNIP MASH `HIGH-CARB DAY`

Serves 6

3 tablespoons coconut oil or good-quality animal fat*
1 kg beef cheek, trimmed and cut into 2 cm cubes
1½ onions, finely chopped
1 carrot, finely chopped
1 celery stalk, finely chopped
3 garlic cloves, finely chopped
200 g beef mince
2 tablespoons Curry Powder (page 172)
600 ml Beef Bone Broth (page 165)
400 g whole peeled tomatoes, crushed (see Note page 66)
2 tablespoons tapioca flour*, mixed with 2 tablespoons water
sea salt and freshly ground black pepper
2 teaspoons lemon juice
1 teaspoon yellow mustard seeds
1 teaspoon brown mustard seeds
2 tablespoons olive oil
2 sprigs Crispy Curry Leaves (page 171)

Parsnip mash
½ garlic bulb, kept intact (break a whole bulb in half with your hands)
2 tablespoons olive oil, plus extra for drizzling
2 large parsnips (about 500 g), peeled and core removed, chopped
½ head of cauliflower (about 600 g), florets cut into 5 cm pieces
1 teaspoon lemon juice
½ teaspoon ground turmeric
1 tablespoon coconut cream

* See Glossary

Heat 2 tablespoons of the coconut oil or animal fat in a large flameproof casserole dish over medium–high heat. Add the beef cubes in batches and cook for 5 minutes, or until browned on all sides. Transfer the meat to a plate and set aside.

Add the remaining oil or fat to the dish, add the onion, carrot, celery and garlic and sauté for 5 minutes until the onion is softened. Reduce the heat to medium, add the mince and, stirring with a wooden spoon to break up the lumps, cook for 3 minutes, or until browned. Stir in the curry powder and cook for a further minute, or until fragrant. Pour in the broth and tomatoes, then return the beef cubes, stir, and bring to a simmer. Cover with the lid, reduce the heat to low and simmer for 3 hours, or until the meat is tender.

Stir the tapioca mixture into the beef and simmer, uncovered, for 30 minutes, or until the sauce is thickened. Season with salt and pepper and allow to cool. Stir in the lemon juice.

Preheat the oven to 180°C (160°C fan-forced).

Place the yellow and brown mustard seeds in a frying pan over medium heat and cook, tossing frequently, until fragrant and toasted. Pour on the olive oil, remove from the heat and set aside.

To start on the parsnip mash, place the garlic on a baking tray, drizzle over some olive oil and roast for 35–40 minutes, or until golden and tender. Meanwhile, bring a large saucepan of salted water to the boil. Add the parsnip and cauliflower and cook for 15–20 minutes until tender. Drain and shake off any excess water. Place the cooked parsnip and cauliflower in a food processor. Cut the roasted garlic in half horizontally and squeeze in the soft garlic flesh. Add the oil, lemon juice, turmeric and coconut cream and process until smooth. Season with salt and pepper to taste.

To assemble the pies, fill six 400 ml capacity ovenproof dishes with the curried meat mixture, leaving 2 cm space at the top. Top with the mash and spread out evenly. Place the dishes on a baking tray and bake for 15–20 minutes, or until the pies are heated through. Spoon the mustard seed oil over the top and finish with the crispy curry leaves.

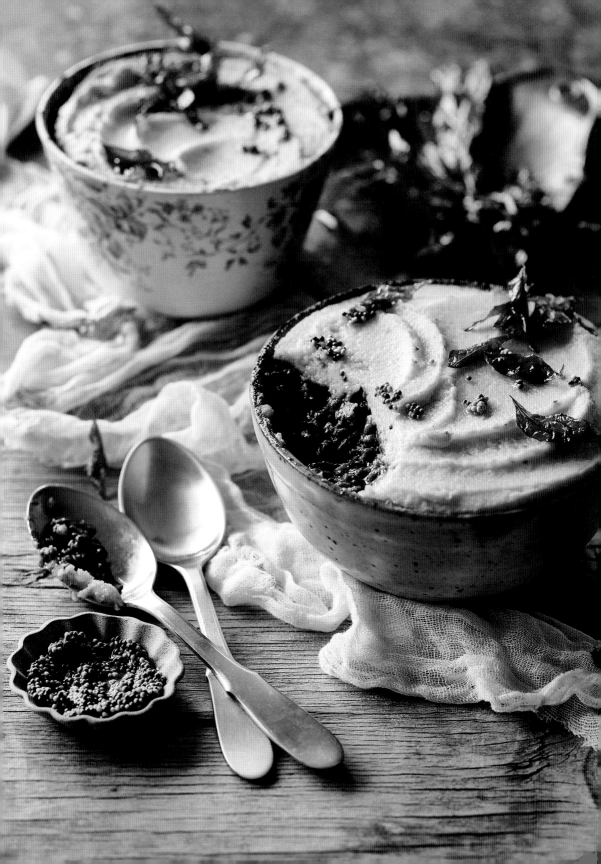

Vitello tonnato is a Piedmontese dish of cold, sliced beef (most often veal but scotch or eye fillet can also be used) covered with a creamy, mayonnaise-like sauce that is enhanced with tuna. Think of this as a very Italian surf and turf! It can be enjoyed as an entree or main or even for breakfast. Also, for a delicious topping or sandwich, try popping it on some keto crackers or bread.

VITELLO TONNATO WITH CRISPY GARLIC AND CAPERS

Serves 3–4 as a starter

2 tablespoons coconut oil or
　good-quality animal fat*
600 g veal or beef fillet, at room
　temperature
sea salt and freshly ground
　black pepper
100 g jarred tuna* in olive oil
　or spring water, drained and
　roughly chopped
3 jarred salted anchovy fillets*,
　rinsed, patted dry and chopped
zest of 1 lemon
1 tablespoon lemon juice
200 g Aioli (page 165)
1 small handful of flat-leaf
　parsley leaves

Crispy garlic and capers
150 ml melted coconut oil
4 garlic cloves, finely sliced
2 tablespoons salted baby capers,
　rinsed well and patted dry

* See Glossary

Preheat the oven to 140°C (120°C fan-forced).

Heat the coconut oil or animal fat in a frying pan over medium–high heat. Season the veal or beef with salt and pepper and sear on each side for 1 minute, or until golden. Place on a baking tray and transfer to the oven to roast for 10 minutes for medium–rare (or cook to your liking). Set aside to rest for 20 minutes, keeping warm.

Place the tuna, anchovies, lemon zest and juice and 150 g of the aioli in a food processor and blend until smooth. Season with salt and pepper and fold through the remaining aioli.

To make the crispy garlic and capers, place the coconut oil and garlic in a saucepan over medium heat and cook until the garlic starts to turn golden. Lift out the garlic with a slotted spoon and drain on paper towel. Using the same pan over medium heat, add the capers and fry until golden. Lift out the capers with a slotted spoon and drain on paper towel.

Slice the veal or beef thinly. Spread some of the tuna aioli onto a serving platter, top with the veal or beef and scatter over the crispy garlic and capers and the parsley leaves. Finish with some salt and a good grind of pepper.

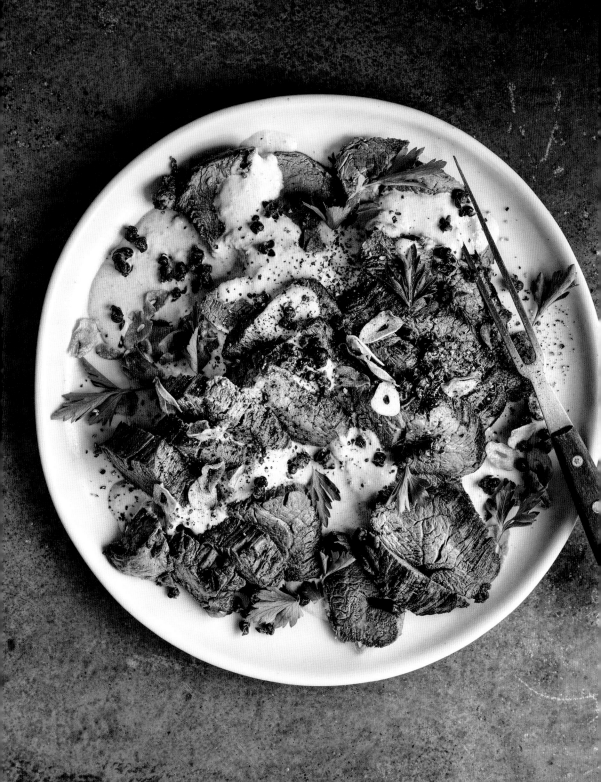

Some days I just love a good steak to break my fast, and it doesn't need to be fancy. I remember being served a simply grilled steak with good-quality salt, olive oil and a lemon cheek in an Italian restaurant 30 years ago. An apprentice chef at the time, I was a little annoyed as I thought not much effort had gone into the meal. Where were all the bells and whistles? Well, from the first bite to the last, it was utterly delicious; the perfect balance of fat, protein, salt and acid. That one dish taught me so much about cooking and has helped shape me into the chef I am today.

SIRLOIN STEAK WITH LEMON, SALT AND OLIVE OIL

Serves 2

1 garlic bulb, halved horizontally
2 x 200 g sirloin steaks
1 tablespoon coconut oil or
   good-quality animal fat*,
   melted
sea salt and freshly ground
   black pepper
1 lemon, halved

* See Glossary

Preheat the oven to 180°C (160°C fan-forced).

Place the garlic on a baking tray and roast for 25–30 minutes, or until golden and tender.

Heat a barbecue grill plate to hot or a large chargrill pan over high heat.

Brush the steaks with the coconut oil or animal fat and season with salt and pepper. Cook the steaks on one side for 3 minutes, or until golden, then flip and cook on the other side for 3 minutes for medium–rare (or cook to your liking). Place the steaks on a plate, loosely cover and rest for 4–6 minutes, keeping warm.

Meanwhile, cook the lemon halves, cut-side down, for 6 minutes, or until charred.

Carve the steak into thick slices and serve with the charred lemon and roasted garlic.

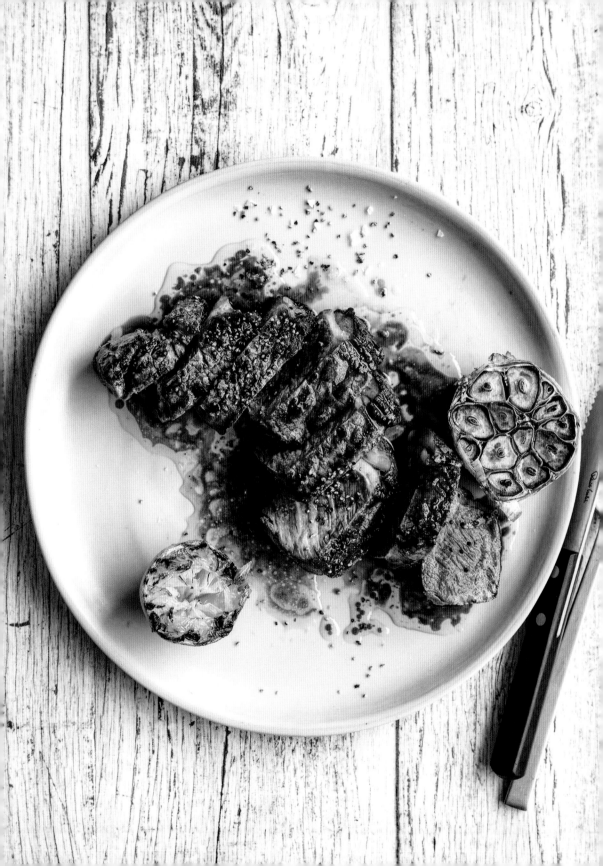

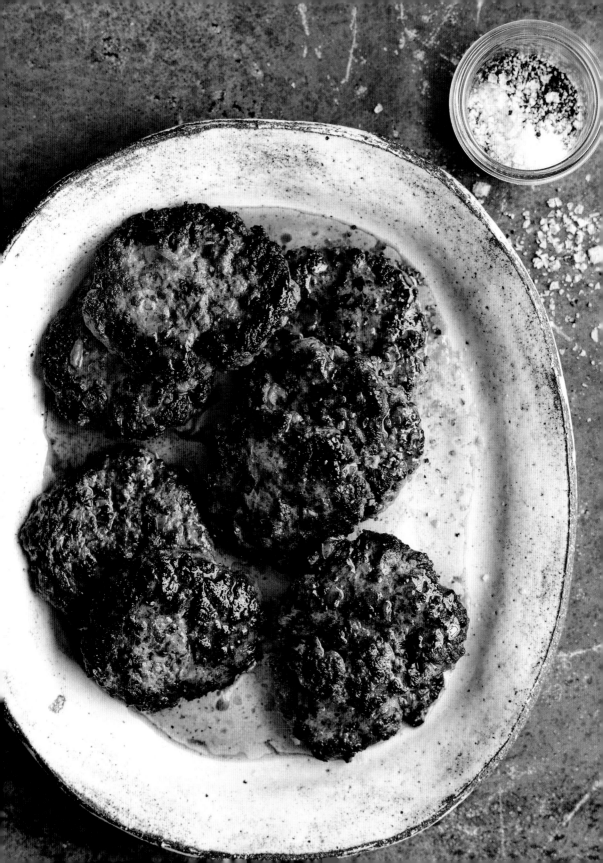

Is there anything better than biting into a juicy flavoursome burger patty? For me, the experience is all about the type of meat, seasoning and spices used, and how the patty is cooked (you want a nice crust on the outside without losing the moisture inside). These patties are a wonderful quick weeknight meal. Eat them straight up, add your favourite salad or veg, or make a burger out of grilled portobello mushrooms, roasted sweet potato or pumpkin, a keto bun or a lettuce wrap.

CLASSIC BEEF BURGERS

Serves 4

coconut oil or good-quality animal fat*, for greasing

Patties
600 g beef mince
1 onion, finely diced
3 garlic cloves, crushed
1 egg
1 tablespoon Worcestershire sauce
¼ teaspoon chilli flakes
2 tablespoons chopped flat-leaf parsley leaves
1 teaspoon dried oregano
1 teaspoon sea salt
1 teaspoon freshly ground black pepper

* See Glossary

Place all the patty ingredients in a large bowl and mix well. Shape into eight patties.

Heat a barbecue hotplate to medium–hot or a large frying pan over medium–high heat. Grease with the coconut oil or animal fat. Add the patties in batches and cook for 3 minutes. Turn the patties and cook on the other side for 2–3 minutes, or until cooked through.

Place the patties on a platter and serve.

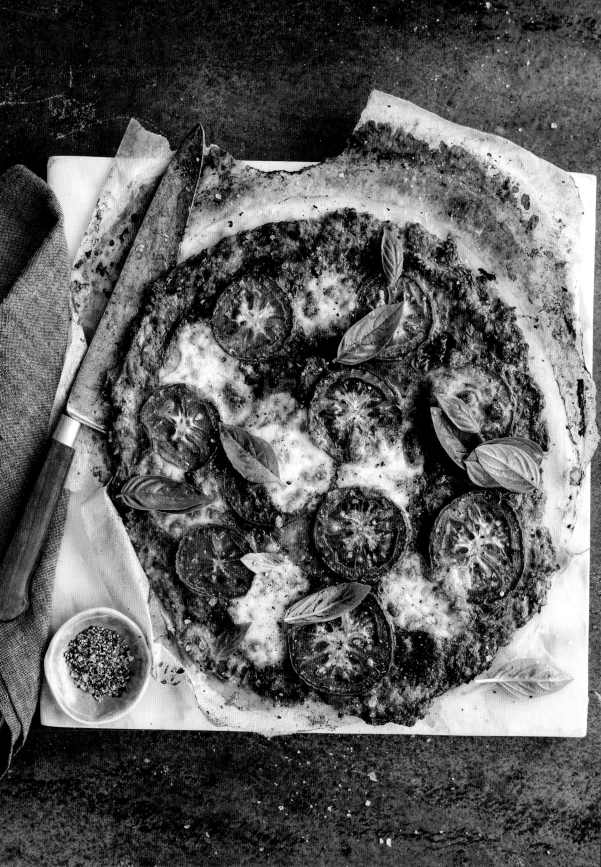

I recently added this meat-based pizza to the menu at a restaurant I am consulting for in Canada, and it has become the owner's favourite. I simply replaced the traditional dough with a burger patty pressed out to resemble a pizza base and, I have to say, it is delicious. Add your favourite pizza toppings, such as olives, anchovies, tomato, fresh or dried herbs and, of course, more meat, such as pepperoni or ham. It is up to you what type of cheese you put on top, but I use a non-dairy one as it works better for my body. Kids love this meatzza – and it is so good for them in so many ways.

MEATZZA

Serves 2–3

coconut oil, for greasing
80 ml (⅓ cup) Pizza Sauce
  (page 175)
6 basil leaves, roughly torn,
  plus extra leaves to serve
1 roma tomato, finely sliced
80 g vegan mozzarella, torn into
  small pieces
sea salt and freshly ground
  black pepper

Base

200 g beef mince
200 g pork mince
1 egg yolk
¼ onion, finely diced
1 garlic clove, finely chopped
1 tablespoon finely chopped
  flat-leaf parsley leaves
½ teaspoon dried oregano
¾ teaspoon sea salt
¼ teaspoon freshly ground
  black pepper

Preheat the oven to 250°C (230°C fan-forced) or the highest temperature setting. Grease a 30 cm pizza tray with a little coconut oil and line with baking paper.

Place all the base ingredients in a bowl and mix until well combined.

Transfer the base mixture to the prepared tray and, using your hands, press it out to evenly cover the surface. Bake for 6–8 minutes until the meat is cooked through. Remove and drain any liquid from the tray.

Spread the pizza sauce evenly over the base. Scatter over the torn basil leaves, then arrange the tomato slices and vegan mozzarella on top. Season with a little salt and pepper.

Return the meatzza to the oven and bake for a further 5–10 minutes until lightly browned.

Use the paper to carefully transfer the meatzza to a chopping board or plate. Cut into slices, scatter over the extra basil leaves and serve.

I never get tired of whipping up this dish. It is probably the one I cook most for my kids' breakfast. I much prefer cooking and eating steak to bacon; I see grass-fed cattle as a healthier option, and a minute steak is quicker to cook. A simple sauce like this chimichurri is all that is needed, or some homemade tomato ketchup (page 179) or your favourite barbecue sauce (page 166 or 178) also fit the bill.

STEAK AND EGGS WITH CHIMICHURRI

Serves 2

4 x 140 g minute steaks
2 tablespoons melted coconut oil
  or good-quality animal fat*
sea salt and freshly ground
  black pepper
4 eggs
Chimichurri (page 171)

* See Glossary

Heat a barbecue hotplate to hot or a large frying pan over high heat.

Brush the steaks with 1 tablespoon of the coconut oil or animal fat and season with a generous amount of salt and pepper. Cook the steaks for 2 minutes, then flip over and cook for 1–2 minutes on the other side for medium–rare (or cook to your liking). Transfer to a plate and allow to rest for 5 minutes, keeping warm.

Heat the remaining oil or fat in a large non-stick frying pan over medium heat. Crack in the eggs and fry for 2–2½ minutes until the egg whites are set (or cook to your liking). Season with salt and pepper.

Serve the steaks on a platter or plates, top each with a fried egg and drizzle over the chimichurri.

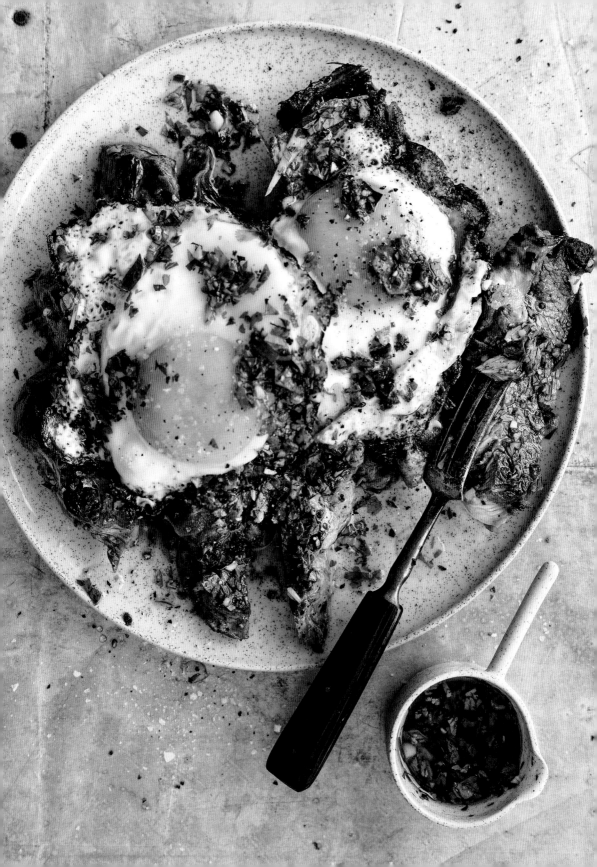

As a kid, Mum making schnitzel was a real treat, and one that I wanted to replicate for this book. The main thing to remember with schnitzel is to balance the healthy fat it is cooked in with some acidity in the form of fresh citrus or vinegar. Here, I have added capers to the sauce, as I find their salty tang completes the dish perfectly.

SCHNITZEL WITH GARLIC AND CAPER SAUCE

Serves 4

4 x 120 g veal escalopes
200 g almond meal, plus extra
  if needed
2 teaspoons onion powder
1 tablespoon finely chopped
  mint leaves
sea salt and freshly ground
  black pepper
60 g (½ cup) tapioca flour*
2 eggs
3 tablespoons almond milk or
  coconut milk
400 ml melted coconut oil or
  good-quality animal fat*
lemon wedges, to serve

Garlic and caper sauce
200 ml melted ghee or
  good-quality animal fat*
8 garlic cloves, finely sliced
3 tablespoons salted baby capers,
  rinsed well and patted dry
2 tablespoons rosemary leaves,
  roughly chopped
2 tablespoons oregano leaves,
  roughly chopped
1 tablespoon lemon juice

* See Glossary

Place the veal between two sheets of baking paper and pound with a meat mallet until evenly flattened.

Combine the almond meal, onion powder and mint in a shallow bowl and mix well. Season with salt and pepper and set aside. Place the tapioca flour in another shallow bowl. In a third bowl, whisk the eggs and almond or coconut milk until well combined.

Working with one piece at a time, dust the pounded veal with the tapioca flour, shaking off any excess. Dip the veal in the egg mixture, then evenly coat with the almond meal mixture.

Heat the coconut oil or animal fat in a large, deep frying pan over medium–high heat until it reaches 160°C. (To test, place a tiny piece of meat in the oil – if the oil starts to bubble around the meat immediately, it is ready.) Shallow-fry the crumbed veal for 1½ minutes on each side until golden and cooked through. Remove from the pan and place on paper towel to drain. Season with a little salt and pepper. Set aside, keeping warm.

Meanwhile, make the garlic and caper sauce. In another frying pan, heat the ghee or fat over medium–high heat. Add the garlic, capers, rosemary and oregano, swirl around the pan and cook for 1–1½ minutes until the garlic starts to colour and the capers are crisp. Pour in the lemon juice, give the sauce another good swirl and season with salt and pepper.

Place the schnitzels on a platter, pour over the garlic and caper sauce and serve with the lemon wedges on the side.

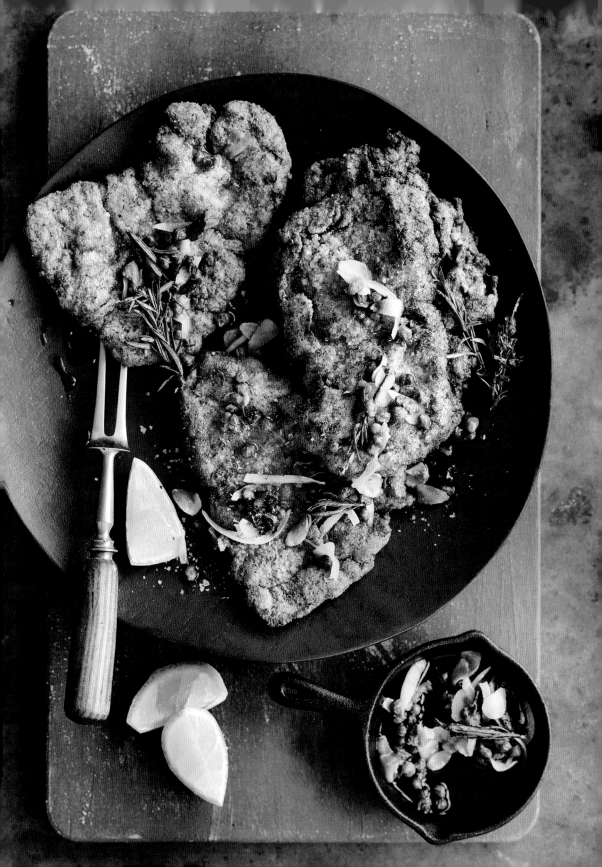

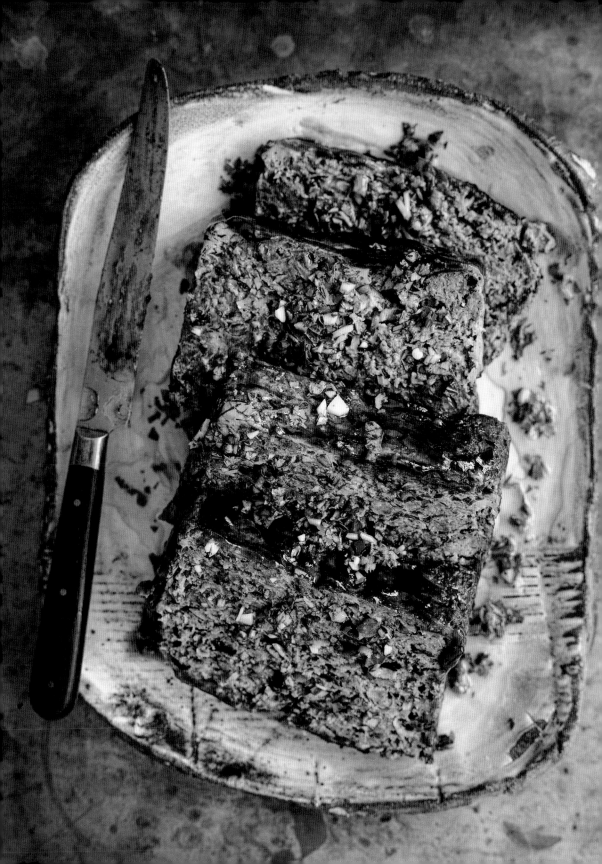

Grass-fed mince meat is a family's most useful and versatile ingredient. We always have some on hand, plus extra in the freezer for whenever we need a great meal. There are so many dishes we can make with mince: nachos, pie fillings, stir-fries, curries, Middle Eastern dishes, burgers, meatballs … and the list goes on. The humble meatloaf is one of the best. We love making it at home, and leftovers are great for breakfast, or school or work lunches the next day.

MEATLOAF

Serves 8

8 rindless streaky bacon rashers
800 g beef mince
3 tablespoons chopped flat-leaf parsley leaves
1 large carrot, grated
100 g English spinach leaves, chopped
200 g field mushrooms, finely chopped
1 large onion, finely diced
2 garlic cloves, crushed
2 eggs, lightly whisked
100 g keto breadcrumbs (keto bread processed into crumbs)
1 teaspoon chilli flakes
1 tablespoon sea salt
1½ teaspoons freshly ground black pepper
3 tablespoons coconut oil or good-quality animal fat*
2 tablespoons Worcestershire sauce
80 ml (⅓ cup) your choice of barbecue sauce (page 166, or 178)
200 g Chimichurri (page 171)

* See Glossary

Preheat the oven to 180°C (160°C fan-forced). Line the base and sides of a 22 cm x 12 cm loaf tin with baking paper, cutting into the corners to fit and allowing the paper to extend 5 cm above the sides.

Line the base and sides of the prepared tin with five slices of bacon (reserve the remaining slices for the top).

Place the mince, parsley, carrot, spinach, mushroom, onion, garlic, egg, breadcrumbs, chilli flakes, salt, pepper, coconut oil or animal fat and Worcestershire sauce in the bowl of a food processor and blitz for 10 seconds until well combined.

Pack the meat mixture into the lined loaf tin, then arrange the remaining bacon slices over the top, tucking them in so they won't overhang the sides. Bake for 30 minutes.

Remove the meatloaf from the oven and baste the top with half the barbecue sauce. Return to the oven and continue to bake for a further 30 minutes, or until cooked through. (To test if it's cooked, insert a thermometer into the meatloaf – it should reach 70°C.) When cool enough to handle, remove the baking paper from the tin by pulling one side – it should slip right out.

Preheat the oven grill to high. Place the meatloaf under the grill for 3–5 minutes to crisp up the skin.

Allow the meatloaf to rest in a warm place for 10 minutes before turning out from the tin. Brush again with the remaining barbecue sauce, then slice and arrange on a platter. Drizzle over the chimichurri and serve.

A good simple marinade to flavour a piece of meat, plus a salad on the side, is all it takes for a terrific meal. I have chosen to use Vietnamese aromatics and a Vietnamese-inspired salad here, but feel free to use whatever spices or aromatics you have on hand. I love the Vietnamese take on this as it is fresh, vibrant, spicy and a little tangy, making you want to go back for more … and more.

VIETNAMESE BEEF SKEWERS

Serves 4

700 g beef eye fillet, cut into 2.5 cm cubes
coconut oil or good-quality animal fat*, for greasing
sea salt and freshly ground black pepper
1 handful of mint leaves
1 handful of coriander leaves
1 handful of Vietnamese mint leaves
1 handful of bean sprouts
3 tablespoons Crispy Shallots (page 172)
3 tablespoons chopped roasted cashews
Vietnamese Pickled Carrot, Cucumber and Daikon (page 179), to serve

Vietnamese dressing

1 tablespoon finely grated ginger
1 tablespoon finely chopped coriander roots and stalks
3 garlic cloves, finely chopped
2 bird's eye chillies, deseeded and chopped
80 ml (⅓ cup) lime juice
2 tablespoons tamari or coconut aminos*
1 tablespoon fish sauce
1 lemongrass stem, pale part only, finely chopped
1 teaspoon sesame oil
80 ml (⅓ cup) extra-virgin olive oil

* See Glossary

Soak 8 bamboo skewers in warm water for 20 minutes before using (or use metal skewers).

Thread 3–4 beef cubes onto each skewer and set aside on a tray.

Combine all the Vietnamese dressing ingredients in a blender and blend until smooth. Set aside.

Pour half the dressing over the skewers, cover and marinate in the fridge for 2 hours or, for best results, overnight. Place the remaining dressing in the fridge.

When you are ready to serve, heat a barbecue grill plate to medium–hot or a large chargrill pan over medium–high heat. Grease with a little coconut oil or animal fat. Season the skewers with salt and pepper and cook for 2 minutes on each side, or until cooked to your liking. Remove from the heat and leave to rest in a warm place for 5 minutes.

Meanwhile, mix the herbs and bean sprouts in a bowl, then arrange on a platter. Add the skewers, spoon over the reserved dressing and sprinkle on the crispy shallots and cashews. Serve with the pickled carrot, cucumber and daikon on the side.

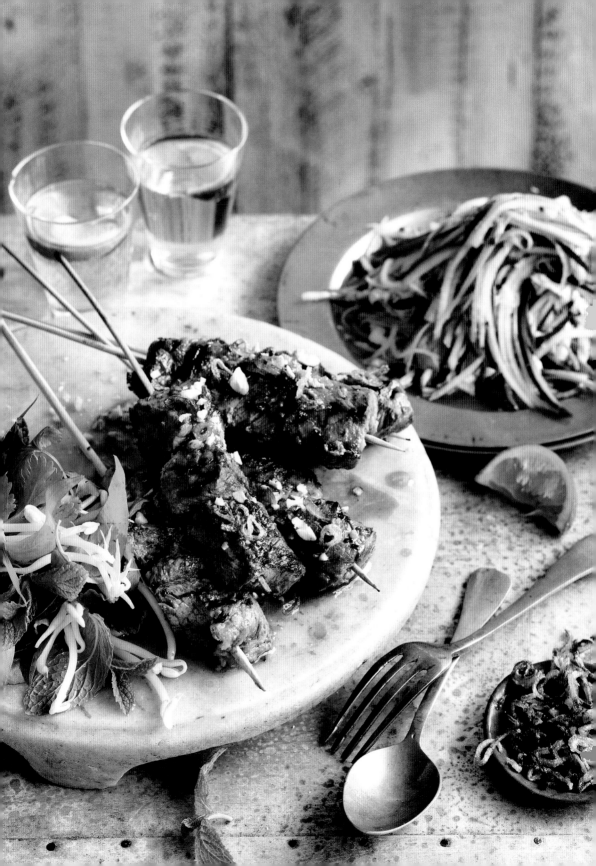

Bordelaise sauce is a classic rich sauce that originates from Bordeaux in France. Made with red wine, demi-glace, bone marrow and shallots, it is very hard to find a better sauce to accompany steak. The richness of the bone marrow and the earthiness of the red wine, shallots and mushrooms is so delicious, you won't know what is better, the steak or the sauce. Let's just say this dish will become a family favourite.

STEAK WITH MUSHROOM BORDELAISE SAUCE

Serves 4

4 x 180–220 g boneless
  rib-eye steaks
2 tablespoons coconut oil or
  good-quality animal fat*
sea salt and freshly ground
  black pepper
1 teaspoon thyme leaves

Mushroom bordelaise sauce
1 x 12 cm piece of beef marrow
  bone, halved lengthways
  (ask your butcher)
2 tablespoons coconut oil or
  good-quality animal fat*
1 French shallot, finely chopped
250 g Swiss brown mushrooms,
  finely sliced
400 ml Red Wine Jus (page 175)

* See Glossary

Preheat the oven to 200°C (180°C fan-forced).

To start the mushroom bordelaise sauce, season the bone marrow with salt, place in a roasting tin and roast in the oven for 15 minutes, or until cooked through. Keep warm.

Heat a barbecue hotplate to medium–hot or a large frying pan over medium–high heat. Brush the steaks with the coconut oil or animal fat and season with a good pinch of salt and pepper. Cook the steaks on one side for 2–3 minutes, then flip and cook for a further 2–3 minutes for medium–rare (or cook to your liking). Transfer to a plate and rest for 4–6 minutes, keeping warm.

Meanwhile, to make the mushroom bordelaise sauce, heat the oil or fat in a large frying pan over medium heat. Add the shallot and sauté for 3 minutes until softened. Add the mushroom and sauté for 5 minutes until softened and lightly golden. Pour in the jus and bring to a simmer. Scoop out the flesh from the marrow bones and toss through the sauce. Taste and season with salt and pepper if needed.

Thickly slice the steak and place on a platter. Pour over the mushroom bordelaise sauce, sprinkle on the thyme and finish with a good grind of pepper.

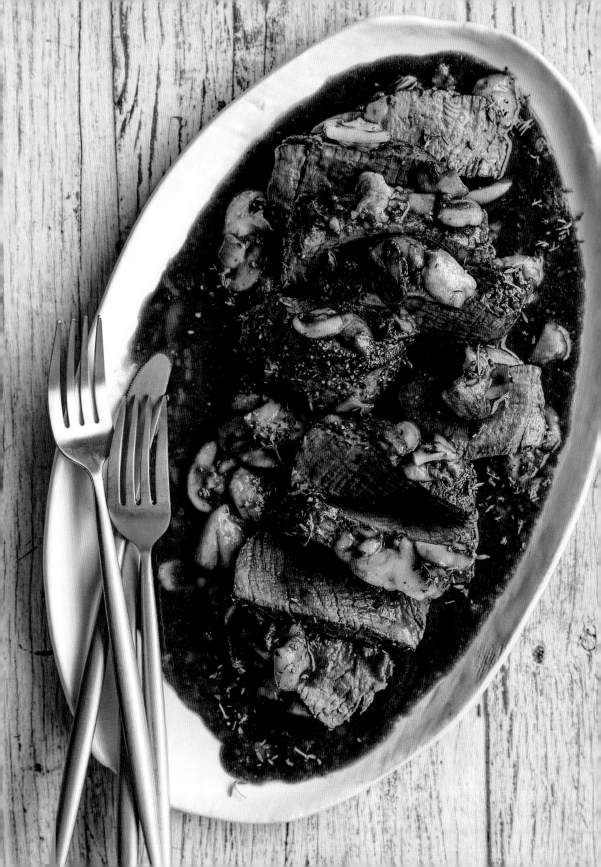

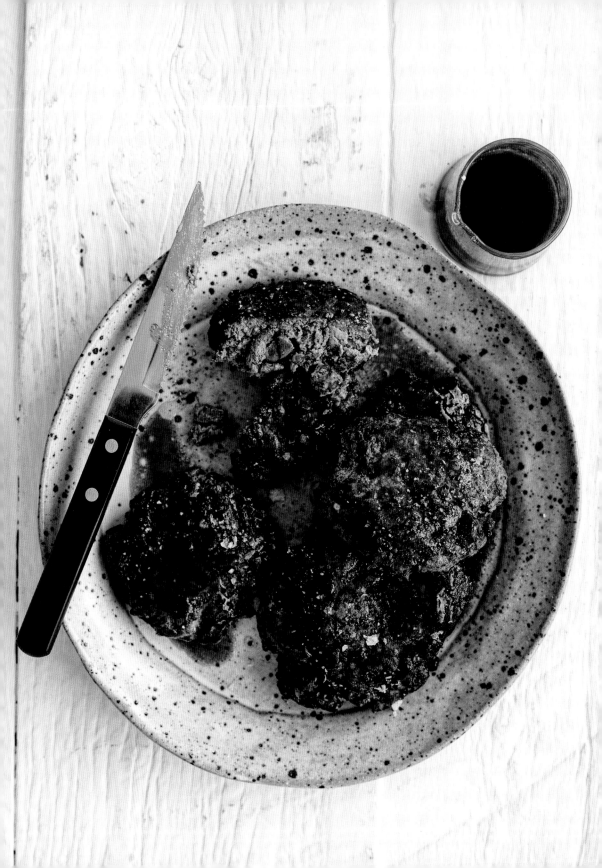

One of the questions I'm often asked is, 'How do I get more offal into my family's diet?' Well, it depends how much you and your family like it – some can tolerate only a small amount until their tastebuds start to appreciate it, whereas others can go all in and have an entire meal of offal. I created these burger patties as a way to gradually introduce offal without anyone knowing it is there. Start off with 5–10 per cent offal and work your way up at your own speed.

OFFAL BURGER PATTIES

Serves 4

1 tablespoon coconut oil or good-quality animal fat*
150 ml your choice of barbecue sauce (page 166 or 178), plus extra to serve
salad of your choice, to serve

Patties
150 g chicken livers
150 g beef heart
80 g bone marrow flesh (ask your butcher)
400 g beef mince
½ onion, finely diced
2 garlic cloves, finely chopped
2 eggs
1 pinch of chilli flakes
1 tablespoon chopped flat-leaf parsley leaves
½ teaspoon dried oregano
1 teaspoon sea salt
1 teaspoon freshly ground black pepper

* See Glossary

To make the patties, rinse the chicken livers under cold water, pat dry with paper towel, trim off any fat, sinew and veins and cut into small pieces. Cut all the fat, vessels, veins and sinew off the beef heart, then chop into cubes. Place the chicken liver, beef heart and marrow flesh in a food processor and pulse a few times until finely minced. Transfer the minced offal meat to a bowl, add the remaining patty ingredients and mix well to combine.

Divide and shape the meat mixture into eight patties.

Heat a barbecue hotplate to medium–hot or a large frying pan over medium–high heat. Brush with the coconut oil or animal fat, add the patties and cook for 3 minutes on one side. Baste with the barbecue sauce, flip over and cook for a further 3 minutes, or until cooked through.

Serve the patties on a platter with salad and the extra barbecue sauce on the side.

Delicious and always rewarding, bolognese is one of the most popular family meals ever. So, how do we make a bolognese sauce even better? Well, to increase the flavour and make it healthier and more satiating, I like to up the fat. Serve this as is or add your favourite vegetable or keto pasta or noodle of choice. Make a big batch: this is amazing reheated the next day for breakfast, with a poached or fried egg on top.

THE ULTIMATE KETO BOLOGNESE

Serves 4–6

2 tablespoons coconut oil or
   good-quality animal fat*
1 onion, chopped
1 carrot, finely diced
1 celery stalk, finely diced
4 garlic cloves, finely chopped
600 g beef mince
2 teaspoons finely chopped
   oregano leaves
200 ml dry red wine (such as
   shiraz) (optional)
3 tablespoons tomato paste
600 g tomato passata
300 ml Brown Chicken Bone
   Broth (page 166)
1 tablespoon chopped basil
   leaves (optional)
1 pinch of chilli flakes (optional)
sea salt and freshly ground
   black pepper

* See Glossary

Heat the coconut oil or animal fat in a large frying pan over medium–high heat. Add the onion, carrot and celery and sauté for 4–5 minutes until softened. Add the garlic and sauté for 1 minute, or until fragrant and starting to brown. Stir in the mince and brown for 5–6 minutes, breaking up the lumps with a wooden spoon.

Add the oregano and wine (if using) to the pan and cook for 4–5 minutes until the wine has almost evaporated. Stir in the tomato paste and cook for 1 minute. Pour in the passata and broth, add the basil and chilli flakes (if using) and season with salt and pepper. Reduce the heat to low and simmer, stirring occasionally, for 40 minutes, or until the meat is cooked through and the sauce is flavoursome and rich.

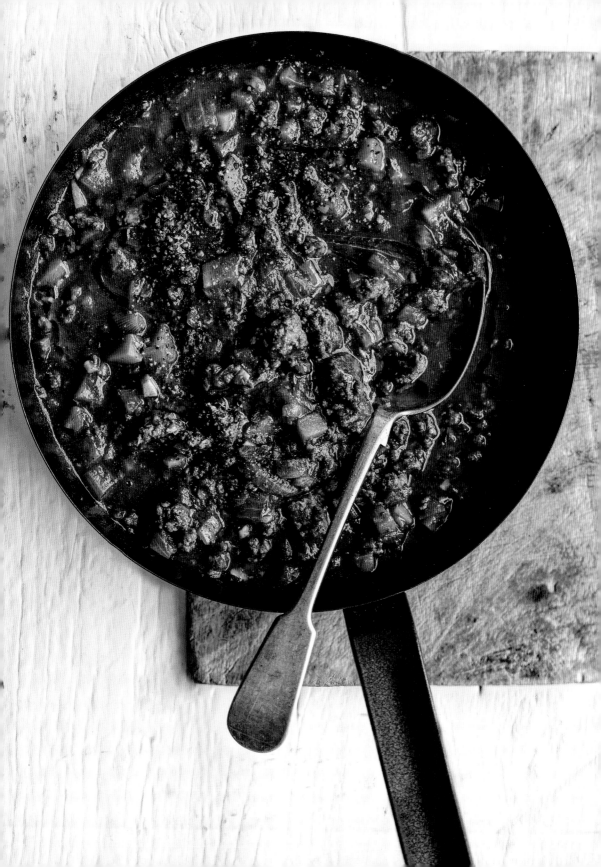

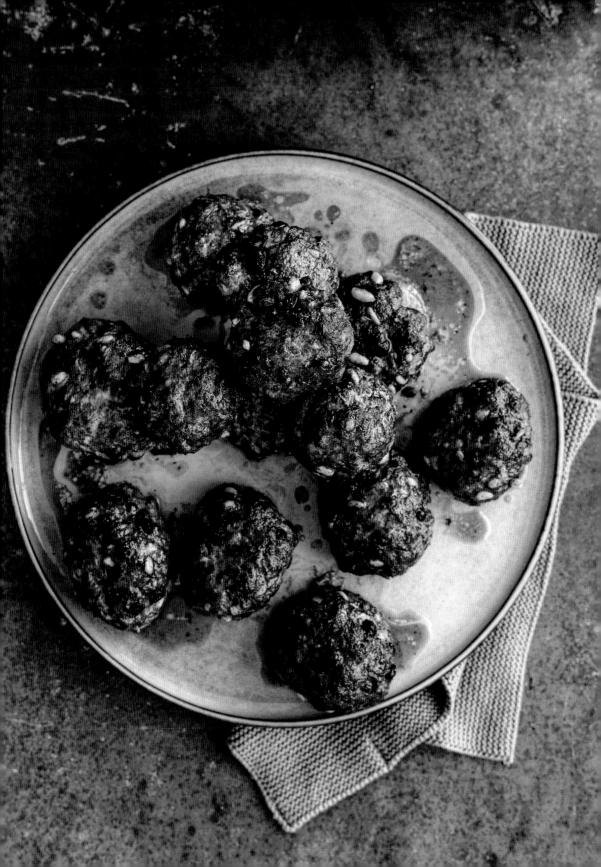

One of my favourite lines in an Australian movie is from *The Castle*, when the family sits down for 'tea' and Darryl asks Sal, 'What do you call these things again?' Her response is, 'Rissoles. Everybody cooks, rissoles, darl.' I laughed so hard when I heard that for the first time.

Rissoles are super delicious and make a wonderful weeknight meal. These ones include pine nuts, and if you are having a higher-carb day, you can add currants for a lovely texture and sweetness, as we have done here. Serve a big platter of these as they are, or add a salad or green veg and some kraut and a dipping sauce.

RISSOLES WITH PINE NUTS AND CURRANTS

HIGH-CARB DAY

Serves 6

3 tablespoons coconut oil or
  good-quality animal fat*
1 onion, finely chopped
1 carrot, finely grated
4 garlic cloves, finely chopped
800 g beef mince
80 g (¾ cup) almond meal
100 g (⅔ cup) currants
130 g pine nuts
3 eggs
3 large handfuls of flat-leaf
  parsley leaves, finely chopped
3 tablespoons tamari or
  coconut aminos*
½ teaspoon chilli flakes
1 tablespoon smoked paprika
1 teaspoon sea salt
1½ teaspoons freshly ground
  black pepper

* See Glossary

Preheat the oven to 200°C (180°C fan-forced). Line a large baking tray with baking paper.

Heat the coconut oil or animal fat in a frying pan over medium heat. Add the onion and sauté for 5 minutes, or until softened. Add the carrot and cook for a further 1 minute until softened. Set aside and allow to cool.

Next, place all the remaining ingredients in a bowl, add the cooled onion mixture and mix well to combine.

Roll the meat mixture into balls about 5 cm in diameter, place on the prepared tray and press down on the balls slightly. Bake the rissoles for 15–18 minutes until cooked through. Serve.

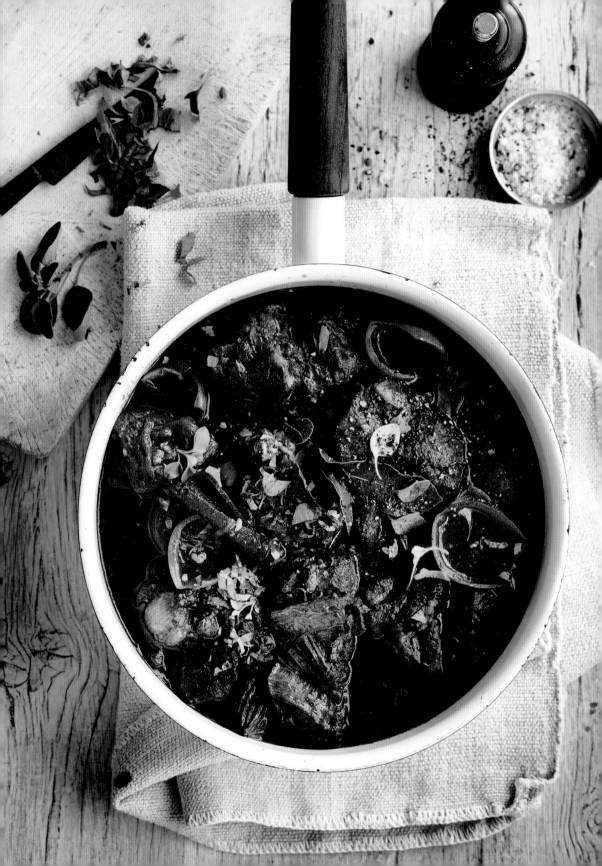

Beef stifado is a wonderful Greek dish with a ton of flavour that's perfect for a weeknight meal when the weather is a bit chilly. You can replace the beef with lamb, pork, chicken or rabbit, but always make more than you think you need because the leftovers are even better the next day.

BEEF STIFADO

Serves 4

8 beef short ribs, bone in
80 ml (⅓ cup) coconut oil or good-quality animal fat*
12 baby onions, halved
sea salt and freshly ground black pepper
2 tablespoons tomato paste
250 ml (1 cup) Beef Bone Broth (page 165), plus extra if needed
400 g whole peeled tomatoes, crushed (see Note page 66)
1 tablespoon roughly chopped oregano leaves

Marinade
4 garlic cloves, finely chopped
4 fresh bay leaves
½ cinnamon stick
½ teaspoon ground allspice
½ teaspoon freshly grated nutmeg
300 ml dry red wine (such as shiraz)
2 tablespoons red wine vinegar

* See Glossary

Place all the marinade ingredients in a large bowl and mix to combine. Add the beef and toss well to evenly coat. Cover and marinate in the fridge for 2 hours or, for best results, overnight.

When you're ready to start cooking, preheat the oven to 120°C (100°C fan-forced).

Heat 2 tablespoons of the coconut oil or animal fat in a large flameproof casserole dish over medium–high heat. Add the onion in batches and cook for 4–6 minutes, turning regularly to get some nice colour on each side. Remove the onion and set aside until needed.

Strain the beef, reserving the marinade.

Add the remaining oil or fat to the dish, then add the beef in batches and sear for about 5 minutes until brown all over. Season with salt and pepper. Remove the meat from the dish and set aside.

Next, add the tomato paste to the dish and cook for 1 minute. Deglaze with the reserved marinade and simmer for 1 minute, or until slightly reduced. Tip in the broth and tomatoes and stir well. Return the meat and onion to the dish and bring to the boil. Cover with the lid and transfer to the oven for 8 hours, or until the meat is tender and falling off the bone. You may need to add more broth or water if the liquid has reduced too much during braising. Remove the bones if you like, but it's fine to leave them in.

Scatter over the oregano and finish with a little salt and a good grind of pepper.

Salisbury steak is not only a great weeknight meal but also comfort food of the highest order. This popular dish, with its origins in Mongolia (via Rome), has been enjoyed in the United States since 1897. It is named after James Salisbury (1823–1905), an American physician and chemist, who advocated for a meat-centred diet to promote health. I have upped the nutritional goodness of the dish by adding a chicken liver gravy and mushrooms. If you are not a fan of liver, then this may be the introduction you have been waiting for. Thanks, Doc!

SALISBURY STEAK WITH MUSHROOM–LIVER GRAVY

Serves 4

3 tablespoons coconut oil or good-quality animal fat*
2 onions, chopped
300 g Swiss brown mushrooms, sliced
2 garlic cloves, finely chopped
2 teaspoons finely chopped thyme leaves
300 ml (2 cups) Red Wine Jus (page 175)
200 ml (2 cups) Chicken Liver Gravy (page 169)
sea salt and freshly ground black pepper

Salisbury steak
600 g beef mince
25 g (¼ cup) keto breadcrumbs (keto bread processed into crumbs)
1 egg
1 tablespoon Worcestershire sauce
1 teaspoon onion powder
½ teaspoon garlic powder
1 teaspoon sea salt
1 teaspoon freshly ground black pepper
1 teaspoon Dijon mustard

* See Glossary

Place all the Salisbury steak ingredients in a food procesor and blend for 10 seconds to combine. Form into four patties.

Heat 2 tablespoons of the coconut oil or animal fat in a large frying pan over medium–high heat. Add the patties and sear for 2 minutes on each side, or until browned. Remove from the pan and set aside.

Add the remaining oil or fat to the pan and reduce the heat to medium. Add the onion and sauté for 8 minutes, or until starting to caramelise. Next, add the mushroom, garlic and thyme and sauté for 4 minutes, or until the mushroom is softened. Mix through the red wine jus and chicken liver gravy and bring back to a simmer. Season with salt and pepper.

Return the Salisbury steak patties to the pan and cook for 1½–2 minutes on each side, or until cooked through. Gradually add a little water if the sauce becomes too thick. Serve.

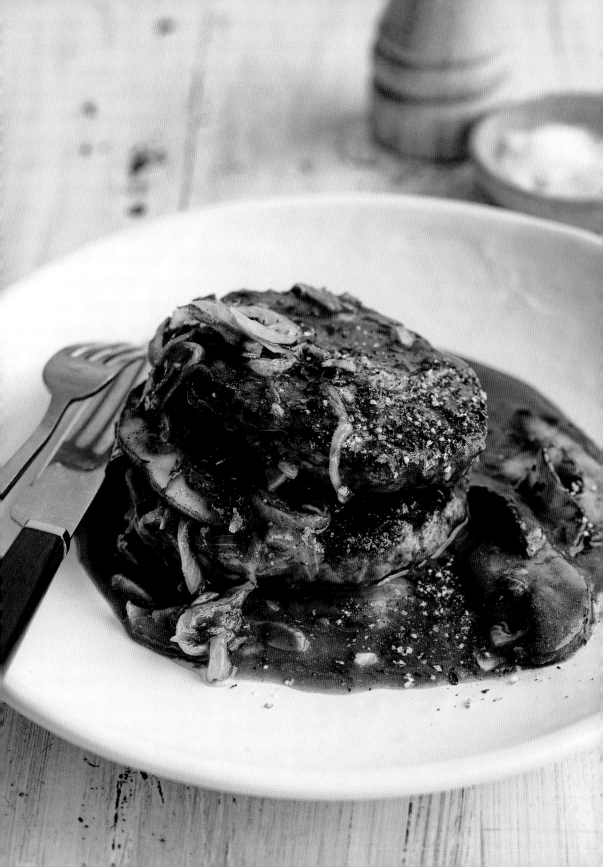

LAMB

Kofta is a type of meatball, meatloaf or skewered meat dish found in many Middle Eastern countries as well as in India, the Balkans and Central Asia. Generally made from minced beef, chicken, lamb or pork mixed with spices, garlic and onion, koftas are grilled over a flame or barbecue. These koftas make for a wonderfully quick weeknight meal, and leftovers come in handy for school or work lunches the next day. Serve yours with sauce and your choice of salad.

LAMB KOFTA

Serves 4

600 g lamb mince
120 g lamb or pork fat, minced (ask your butcher)
3 garlic cloves, finely chopped
2 teaspoons ground cumin
2 teaspoons dried mint
2 teaspoons dried oregano
2 teaspoons sweet paprika
½ teaspoon chilli flakes
2 teaspoons pomegranate molasses*, plus extra to serve
sea salt and freshly ground black pepper
olive oil, for brushing
1 handful of mint leaves

Spiced coconut yoghurt
200 g coconut yoghurt
½ teaspoon ground cumin
2 tablespoons pomegranate molasses*
extra-virgin olive oil, for drizzling

* See Glossary

Soak eight bamboo skewers in warm water for 20 minutes (or use metal skewers).

Combine the lamb mince, lamb or pork fat, garlic, cumin, dried mint and oregano, paprika, chilli flakes, pomegranate molasses and some salt and pepper in a bowl and mix thoroughly.

Divide the lamb mixture into eight portions, then shape each portion around a skewer. Place the skewers on a tray, cover and refrigerate for 30 minutes.

Heat a barbecue hotplate to medium or a large frying pan over medium heat and brush with a little olive oil. Add the skewers and cook for 3½ minutes, then turn and cook for a further 3½ minutes, or until cooked through.

To make the spiced coconut yoghurt, combine the coconut yoghurt and cumin and season with salt and pepper. Spoon into a small bowl and drizzle over the pomegranate molasses and a little extra-virgin olive oil.

Arrange the lamb skewers on a platter and scatter over the mint leaves. Serve with the spiced coconut yoghurt on the side. If you like, you can drizzle a little extra pomegranate molasses over the skewers.

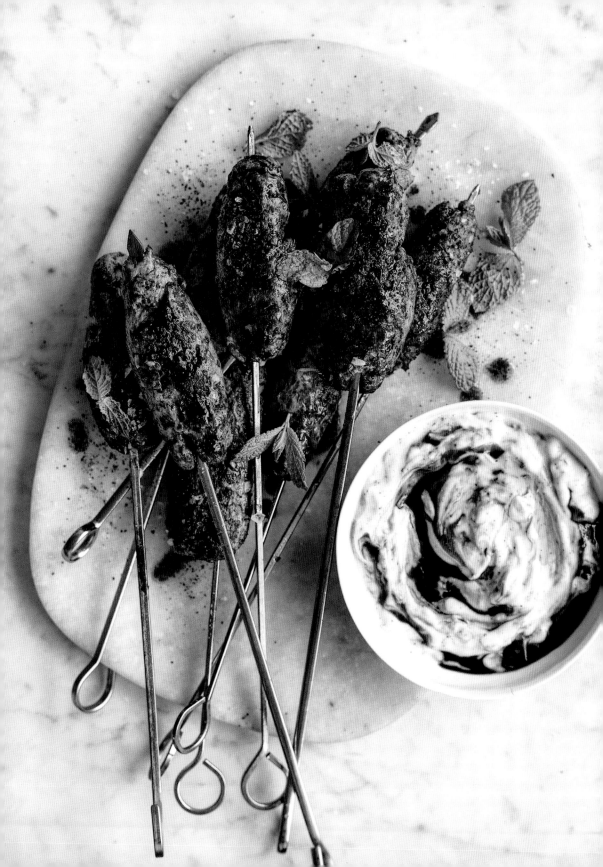

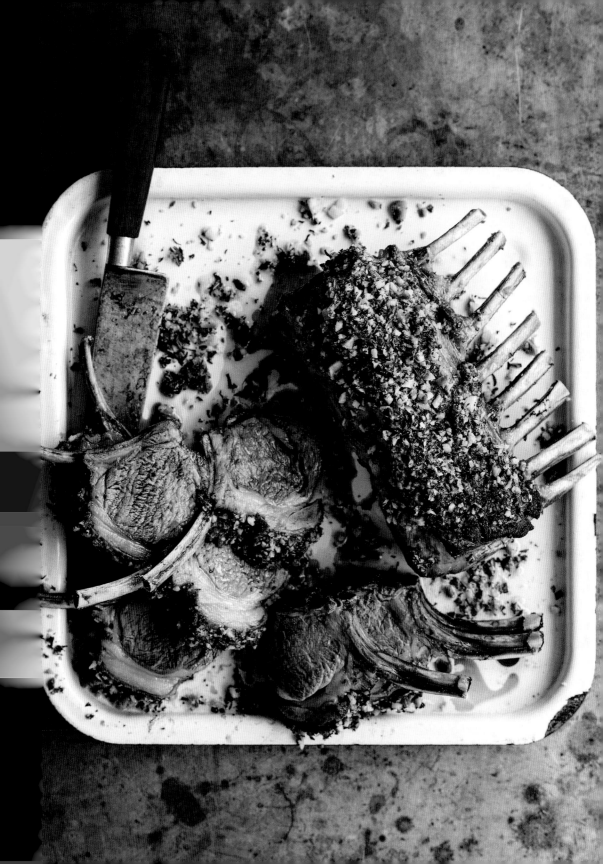

Often the classic dishes are the ones I go back to time and time again. Take, for instance, this crusted lamb rack; I really am pushed to find a better recipe. This dish has stood the test of time because it showcases an amazing cut of lamb without overpowering its wonderful flavour. Admittedly, lamb racks are very expensive these days, so I see this as something to enjoy on special occasions. Serve with a side of veg or salad, or go full carnivore and enjoy the meat with no distractions.

HERB AND MUSTARD LAMB RACKS

Serves 4–6

6 garlic cloves, finely chopped

3 tablespoons nutritional yeast*

1 large handful of flat-leaf parsley leaves, finely chopped

3 tablespoons finely chopped mint leaves

2 teaspoons finely chopped rosemary leaves

80 ml (⅓ cup) melted coconut oil or good-quality animal fat*

sea salt and freshly ground black pepper

2 x 8-rib lamb racks, French trimmed (ask your butcher), at room temperature

3 tablespoons Dijon mustard

* See Glossary

Preheat the oven to 200°C (180°C fan-forced).

Place the garlic, nutritional yeast, parsley, mint, rosemary and 2 tablespoons of the coconut oil or animal fat in a bowl, season with salt and pepper and stir well to combine.

Season the lamb rack with salt and pepper.

Heat the remaining oil or fat in a large frying pan over medium–high heat. Add the lamb in batches and cook for 3–4 minutes on each side, or until browned all over. Transfer the lamb, fat-side up, to a large baking tray.

Spread the mustard over the fatty side of the lamb racks. Divide the herb mixture in two, then spread and pat each portion over the mustard coating on each lamb rack.

Roast the lamb racks for 20–25 minutes for medium–rare (or cook to your liking). Allow to rest for 10 minutes, keeping warm.

Cut each lamb rack into individual cutlets to serve.

'Shut the gate' is one of the funniest ways to express when something is so fantastic that there is nothing left to say on the matter. Well, I reckon this lamb rib dish is one of the best I have ever had the pleasure of cooking and eating; so, yeah . . . shut the damn gate! In all seriousness, though, ribs are the tastiest cut of lamb as they have an amazing layer of fat on top of the meat. When cooked slowly in spices until the meat is falling off the bone, and finished with a zingy chermoula, not much can top them.

LAMB RIBS WITH CHERMOULA

Serves 4

1.5 kg lamb ribs
3 tablespoons lard or other
    good-quality animal fat*
sea salt and freshly ground
    black pepper

Chermoula
1 large handful of coriander
    leaves, chopped
1 large handful of flat-leaf parsley
    leaves, chopped
1 large handful of mint leaves,
    chopped
2 garlic cloves, chopped
1½ teaspoons ground cumin
1½ teaspoons ground coriander
1 teaspoon smoked paprika
½ long red chilli, deseeded
    and chopped
3 tablespoons lemon juice
125 ml (½ cup) olive oil
sea salt and freshly ground
    black pepper

* See Glossary

To make the chermoula, combine the herbs, garlic, spices, chilli and lemon juice in a food processor and process to a paste. With the motor running, drizzle in the olive oil and process until smooth. Season with salt and pepper to taste.

Preheat the oven to 150°C (130°C fan-forced).

Rub the ribs with the fat and sprinkle with a generous amount of salt and pepper.

Heat a large flameproof casserole dish over medium–high heat. Add the ribs in batches and seal on all sides for 4–5 minutes until browned.

Return all the ribs to the dish, cover with the lid and roast in the oven for 3 hours, or until the meat is tender and falling off the bone.

Cut the ribs into pieces, drizzle over the chermoula and serve.

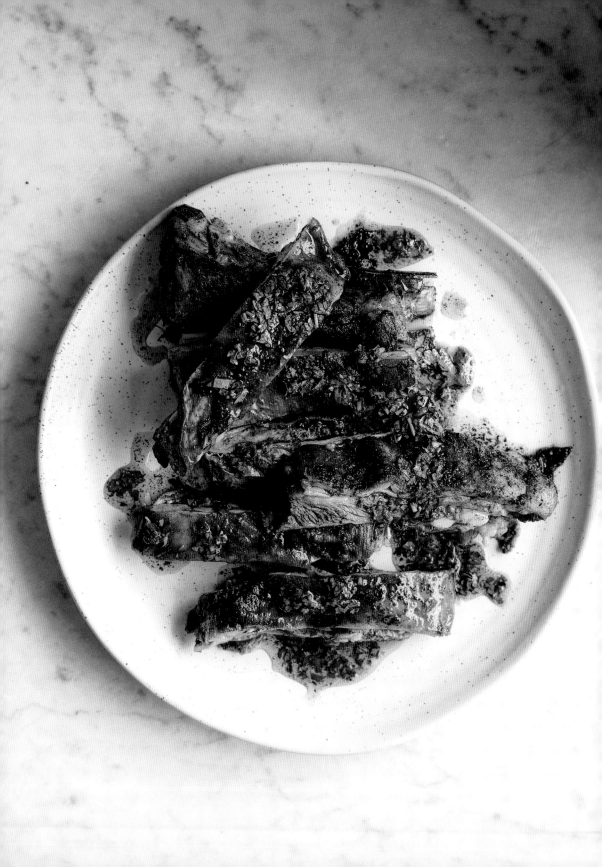

Sometimes a hearty piece of meat needs a hearty sauce to match – and this West Indian lamb shank curry pairs the two perfectly. Secondary cuts of meat like shanks need to be cooked long and slow to add flavour and give the fat and connective tissue time to become tender. A winner in every sense of the word, this is curry delicious served with cauliflower rice (page 167).

WEST INDIAN LAMB SHANK CURRY

Serves 4

4 x 300 g lamb shanks, French trimmed (ask your butcher), at room temperature
100 ml melted coconut oil or good-quality animal fat*
40 g (⅓ cup) Curry Powder (page 172)
sea salt and freshly ground black pepper
1 onion, finely chopped
1 carrot, finely chopped
1 celery stalk, finely chopped
½ habanero chilli, deseeded and finely chopped
4 garlic cloves, crushed
1 tablespoon finely grated ginger
400 ml coconut milk
500 ml (2 cups) Beef Bone Broth (page 165)
5 vine-ripened tomatoes, chopped
1 teaspoon thyme leaves
2 fresh bay leaves
1½ zucchini, sliced
1 handful of herbs (such as dill fronds and coriander leaves)
lime wedges, to serve

* See Glossary

Pat the lamb shanks dry with paper towel and transfer to a large bowl. Drizzle with 2 tablespoons of the coconut oil or animal fat, then sprinkle over half of the curry powder and season with a generous amount of salt and pepper. Toss the lamb shanks gently to evenly coat with the oil and seasoning. Cover and marinate in the fridge for 1 hour.

Preheat the oven to 150°C (130°C fan-forced).

Heat 1 tablespoon of the oil or fat in a large flameproof casserole dish over medium–high heat. Add the shanks in batches and brown until golden, about 1 minute on each side. Do not overcrowd the pan. Remove the shanks from the dish and set aside. Wipe the dish clean.

Heat the remaining oil or fat in the dish, add the onion, carrot, celery and chilli and sauté for about 5 minutes until just starting to colour. Stir in the garlic, ginger and the remaining curry powder, mix well with a wooden spoon and continue to sauté for 1–2 minutes.

Return the shanks to the dish, add the coconut milk, broth, tomato, thyme and bay leaves and stir to combine. Season with salt and pepper. Bring to the boil, cover with the lid and transfer to the oven. Braise for 3 hours, then stir in the zucchini, cover and cook for a further 1 hour, or until the meat is falling off the bone. Season with salt and pepper.

Skim the layer of fat off the top of the curry if needed. Scatter over the herbs and serve with the lime wedges.

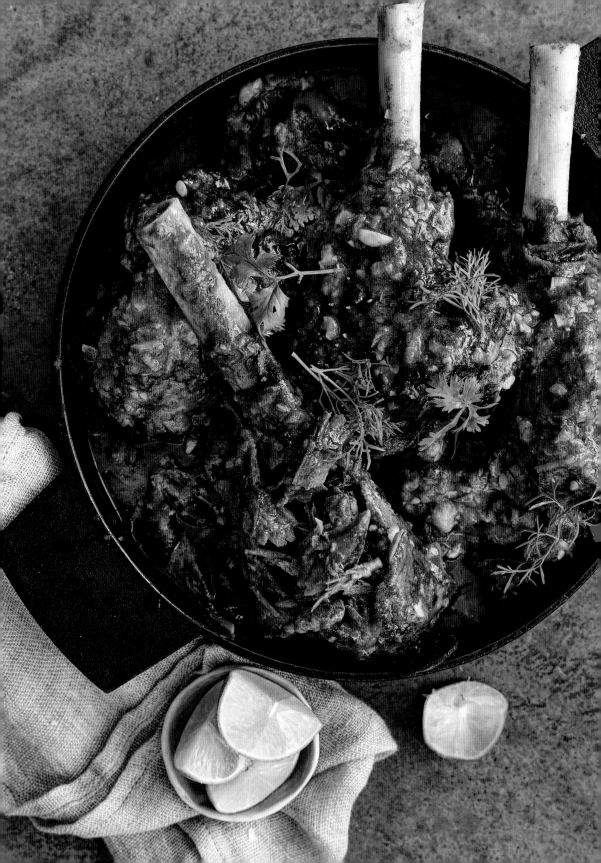

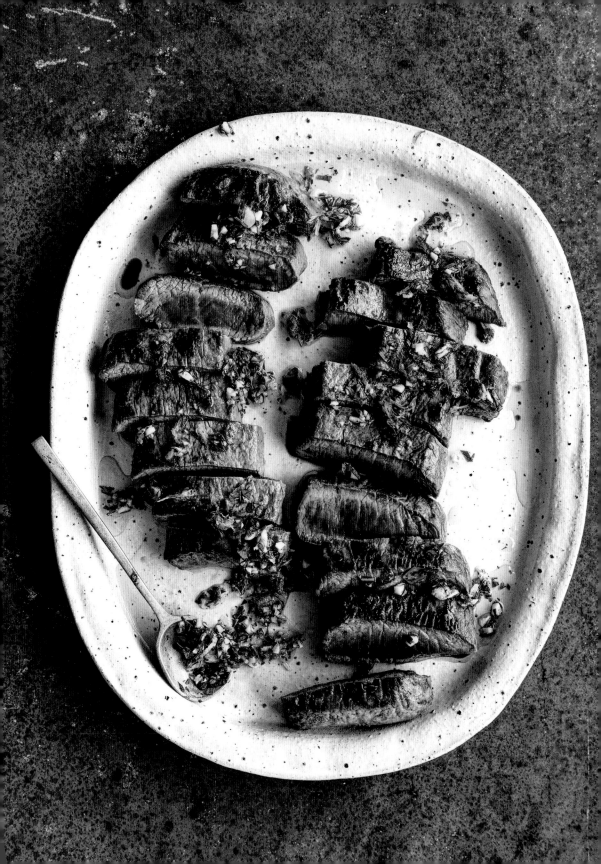

Gremolata is an Italian herb mixture served with grilled or roasted meats. It is made up of lemon zest (and sometimes the juice), garlic and fresh herbs – such as parsley and mint. I like to turn it into a sauce with the addition of some extra-virgin olive oil. This simple dish uses lamb backstrap, but you could also try lamb loin or chops or even sausages for a wonderful lunch or dinner.

LAMB BACKSTRAP WITH GREMOLATA SAUCE

Serves 4

2 x 350 g lamb backstraps, trimmed, at room temperature
2 tablespoons coconut oil or good-quality animal fat*
sea salt and freshly ground black pepper

Gremolata sauce
2 large handfuls of flat-leaf parsley leaves, finely chopped
2 garlic cloves, finely chopped
finely grated zest and juice of 1 lemon, or to taste
120 ml extra-virgin olive oil
sea salt and freshly ground black pepper

* See Glossary

Combine all the gremolata sauce ingredients in a small bowl and set aside for 15 minutes to allow the flavours to develop. Taste and season with more salt and pepper if needed.

Brush the lamb with the coconut oil or animal fat and season with salt and pepper.

Heat a large frying pan over medium–high heat. Add the lamb and cook for 3 minutes on each side for medium–rare (or cook to your liking). Transfer to a plate and allow to rest for 5 minutes, keeping warm.

Slice the lamb and arrange on a platter, drizzle over the gremolata sauce and serve.

One of the more unusual flavour combinations I was introduced to when I started my chef apprenticeship about 30 years ago was the marriage of anchovy and lamb. The salty nature of anchovies works so well with lamb, that I have used this combination in many ways since that first encounter. Try this classic surf and turf for yourself, I know you'll be convinced.

LAMB CHOPS WITH ANCHOVY AIOLI

Serves 4

4 x 180 g lamb forequarter chops
sea salt and freshly ground
  black pepper
1 pinch of dried mint
½ teaspoon ground cumin
3 tablespoons coconut oil or
  good-quality animal fat*

Anchovy aioli
6 jarred salted anchovy fillets*,
  rinsed and patted dry,
  finely chopped
1 tablespoon finely chopped
  dill fronds
1 tablespoon finely chopped
  flat-leaf parsley leaves
250 g (1 cup) Aioli (page 165)
sea salt and freshly ground
  black pepper

* See Glossary

Place all the anchovy aioli ingredients in a bowl and mix to combine. Taste and season with more salt and pepper if needed.

Season the lamb chops with salt and pepper and sprinkle over the dried mint and cumin.

Heat the coconut oil or animal fat in a large frying pan over medium–high heat. Add the lamb and cook, turning occasionally, for 6–7 minutes for medium–rare (or cook to your liking). Transfer to a plate and allow to rest for 5 minutes, keeping warm.

Serve the lamb chops with the anchovy aioli.

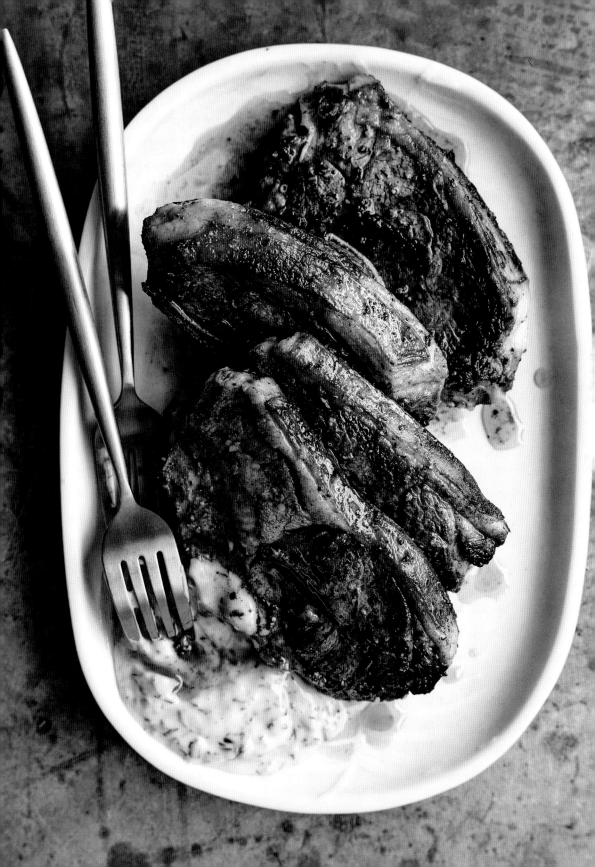

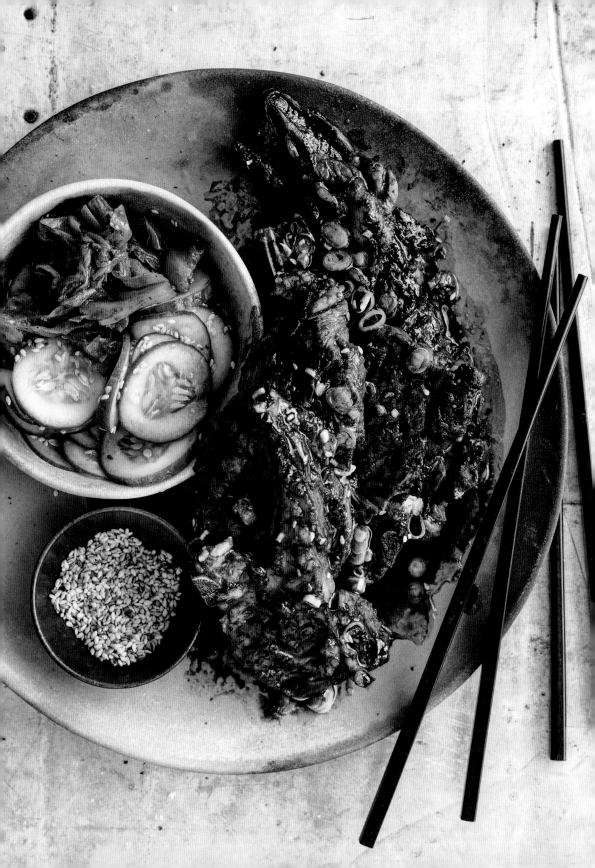

There is something so tantalising about sitting down to a plate of lamb chops that always gets me licking my lips in anticipation of the feast I'm about to enjoy. To add to the experience and make it even more pleasurable, here the chops are prepared Kalbi-style, marinated and served with the sauce. This would have to be one of my all-time favourite meals.

BARBECUED KOREAN KALBI LAMB CHOPS HIGH-CARB DAY

Serves 4

6 forequarter lamb chops, cut in half lengthways
2 tablespoons coconut oil or good-quality animal fat*
sea salt and freshly ground black pepper
kimchi, to serve

Marinade
8 garlic cloves, finely chopped
1½ tablespoons finely grated ginger
125 ml (½ cup) tamari or coconut aminos*
140 ml kombucha
90 g (¼ cup) honey
2 tablespoons sesame oil
2 spring onions, finely chopped

Seasoned cucumber
2 Lebanese cucumbers, finely sliced
1 teaspoon sea salt
1 tablespoon apple cider vinegar
1 teaspoon sesame seeds, toasted, plus 1 tablespoon extra to serve

* See Glossary

Combine all the marinade ingredients in a bowl large enough to fit the lamb in a single layer. Add the lamb and turn to coat thoroughly. Cover and marinate in the fridge for 4 hours or, for best results, overnight.

When you're ready to cook the lamb, heat a barbecue grill plate to medium–hot or a chargrill pan over medium–high heat and brush with the coconut oil or animal fat. Remove the lamb from the bowl (reserve the marinade), season with salt and pepper and cook for 3 minutes on each side, or until browned. Allow to rest for a few minutes, keeping warm.

Pour the reserved marinade into a small saucepan and bring to a simmer. Cook for 5 minutes, or until the sauce coats the back of a spoon.

To make the seasoned cucumber, toss the cucumber and salt together in a large bowl and set aside for 5 minutes. Gently squeeze the cucumber with your hands to remove any excess liquid. Transfer to another bowl, stir in the vinegar and sprinkle over the sesame seeds.

Place the lamb chops on serving plates and spoon over the sauce. Serve with the seasoned cucumber, kimchi and extra sesame seeds on the side.

BASICS

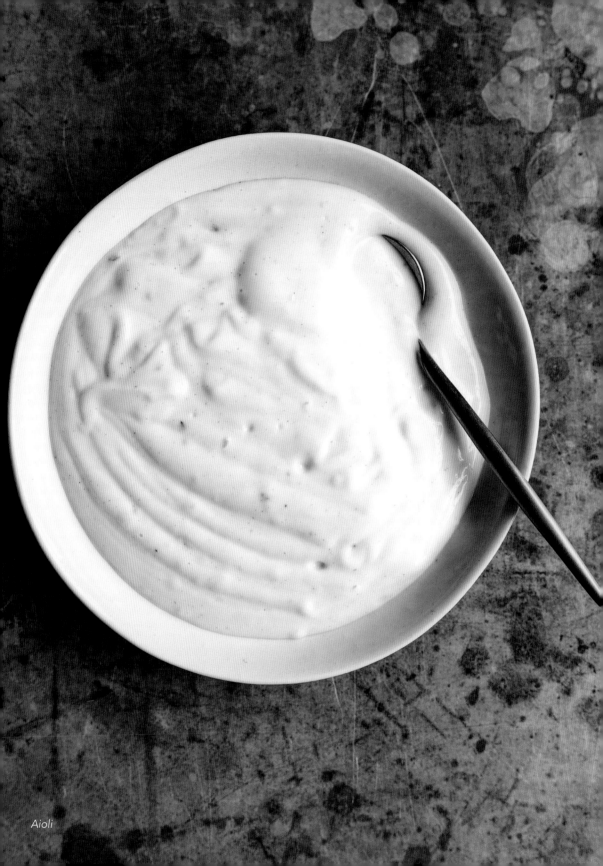

Aioli

AIOLI

Makes 470 g

6 roasted garlic cloves
4 egg yolks
2 teaspoons Dijon mustard
2 teaspoons apple cider vinegar
1½ tablespoons lemon juice
420 ml (1⅔ cups) olive oil
sea salt and freshly ground black pepper

Combine the garlic, egg yolks, mustard, vinegar, lemon juice and olive oil in a glass jug. Using a hand-held blender, blend, working the blade from the bottom of the jug slowly to the top, until thick and creamy. Alternatively, place the garlic, egg yolks, mustard, vinegar and lemon juice in a food processor and process until combined. With the motor running, slowly pour in the oil in a thin, steady stream and process until the aioli is thick and creamy. Season with salt and pepper. Store in an airtight container in the fridge for up to 5 days.

BEEF BONE BROTH

Makes 4 litres

2 kg beef knuckle and marrow bones
1 calf's foot, chopped into pieces (optional)
3 tablespoons apple cider vinegar
1.5 kg meaty beef rib or neck bones
3 onions, roughly chopped
3 carrots, roughly chopped
3 celery stalks, roughly chopped
2 leeks, white part only, roughly chopped
3 thyme sprigs
2 fresh bay leaves
1 teaspoon black peppercorns, crushed
1 garlic bulb, halved horizontally
2 large handfuls of flat-leaf parsley stalks

Place the knuckle and marrow bones and calf's foot (if using) in a stockpot, add the vinegar and pour in 5 litres of cold water, or enough to cover. Set aside to stand for 1 hour.

Preheat the oven to 180°C (160°C fan-forced).

Place the meaty bones in a large roasting tin and roast for 30–40 minutes until well browned. Add the meaty bones to the stockpot along with the vegetables.

Pour the fat from the roasting tin into a saucepan, add 1 litre of water, place over high heat and bring to a simmer, stirring with a wooden spoon to loosen any coagulated juices. Add this liquid to the bones and vegetables. Add additional water, if necessary, to cover the bones and vegetables; the liquid should come no higher than 2 cm below the rim of the pot, as the volume will expand slightly during cooking.

Bring the broth to the boil, skimming off the scum that rises to the top. Reduce the heat to low and add the thyme, bay leaves, peppercorns and garlic. Simmer for 8–12 hours, adding the parsley in the last 10 minutes.

Strain the broth through a fine sieve into a large container. Cover and cool in the fridge. Remove the congealed fat that rises to the top (it is a fantastic, stable cooking fat) and store it in a glass container in the fridge for up to 2 weeks – use it for frying and sautéing. Transfer the gelatinous broth to smaller airtight containers and store in the fridge for up to 4 days or freeze for up to 3 months.

BROCCOLI RICE

Serves 4

2 heads of broccoli (about 400 g each),
    florets and stalk roughly chopped
2 tablespoons coconut oil
sea salt and freshly ground black pepper

Place the broccoli in a food processor and pulse into tiny pieces that look like rice.

Melt the coconut oil in a large frying pan over medium heat. Add the broccoli and cook, stirring occasionally, for 4–6 minutes until softened. Season with salt and pepper. The rice is best eaten straight away, but can be stored in an airtight container in the fridge for up to 4 days.

BROWN CHICKEN BONE BROTH

Makes 4 litres

3 kg bony chicken parts (such as necks,
  breastbones and wings)
2–4 chicken feet
2 tablespoons apple cider vinegar
1 large onion, roughly chopped
2 carrots, roughly chopped
3 celery stalks, roughly chopped
1 leek, white part only, roughly chopped
1 garlic bulb, broken into cloves
1 tablespoon black peppercorns, lightly crushed
2 large handfuls of flat-leaf parsley stalks
2 fresh bay leaves

Preheat the oven to 200°C (180°C fan-forced).

Place the chicken bones and feet in a couple of
large roasting tins and roast for 30–40 minutes
until well browned.

Place the roasted chicken bones and feet in
a stockpot. Add 5 litres of cold water, the vinegar,
onion, carrot, celery, leek, garlic and peppercorns.
Place over medium–high heat and bring to the
boil, skimming off the scum that forms on the
surface. Reduce the heat to low and simmer for
8–12 hours, adding the parsley and bay leaves
in the last 10 minutes. The longer you cook the
broth the more the flavour develops.

Allow the broth to cool slightly, then strain
through a fine sieve into a large storage container.
Cover and cool in the fridge. Remove the
congealed fat that rises to the top (it is a fantastic,
stable cooking fat) and store in a glass container
in the fridge for up to 2 weeks – use it for frying
and sautéing. Transfer the gelatinous broth to
smaller airtight containers and store in the fridge
for up to 4 days or freeze for up to 3 months.

CAROLINA-STYLE BARBECUE SAUCE

Makes 400 ml

125 ml (½ cup) apple cider vinegar
2 tablespoons Dijon mustard
3 tablespoons Worcestershire sauce
2 tablespoons honey
2 garlic cloves, finely grated
½ teaspoon sea salt
1 teaspoon chilli powder
1 teaspoon smoked paprika
¼ teaspoon freshly ground black pepper
1½ teaspoons tapioca flour*, mixed with
  1 tablespoon water
125 ml (½ cup) Smoked Lard (page 176)
  or melted lard

* See Glossary

Place the vinegar, mustard, Worcestershire sauce,
honey, garlic, salt and spices in a small saucepan
and whisk well to combine. Place over medium–
low heat and simmer, stirring occasionally, for
10 minutes to allow the flavours to develop.

Whisk the tapioca mixture into the simmering
sauce and continue to whisk until the sauce
thickens enough to coat the back of a spoon.
Remove from the heat, then whisk in the lard.

Taste and season with a little more salt and
pepper if needed. Allow to cool. Store in an
airtight container in the fridge for up to 3 weeks.

TIP

This sauce is best served at room temperature,
as the lard causes it to solidify when refrigerated.
Gently warm the sauce on the stovetop and whisk
until smooth before using.

CAULIFLOWER AND BROCCOLI RICE

Serves 4–6

½ head of cauliflower (about 500 g), florets
   and stalk roughly chopped
1 head of broccoli (about 300 g), florets and
   stalk roughly chopped
2 tablespoons coconut oil
sea salt and freshly ground black pepper

Place the cauliflower and broccoli in a food
processor and pulse into tiny pieces that look
like rice.

Melt the coconut oil in a large frying pan over
medium heat. Add the cauliflower and broccoli
and cook, stirring occasionally, for 4–6 minutes
until softened. Season with salt and pepper. The
rice is best eaten straight away, but can be stored
in an airtight container in the fridge for up to
4 days.

CAULIFLOWER RICE

Serves 4–6

1 head of cauliflower (about 1 kg), florets
   and stalk roughly chopped
2 tablespoons coconut oil
sea salt and freshly ground black pepper

Place the cauliflower in a food processor and
pulse into tiny pieces that look like rice.

Melt the coconut oil in a large frying pan over
medium heat. Add the cauliflower and cook,
stirring occasionally, for 3–4 minutes until
softened. Season with salt and pepper. The rice is
best eaten straight away, but can be stored in an
airtight container in the fridge for up to 4 days.

CHICKEN JUS

Makes 650 ml

2 French shallots, chopped
6 thyme sprigs
300 ml dry white wine (such as sauvignon blanc)
1 tablespoon Dijon mustard
3 litres Brown Chicken Bone Broth (page 166)
1½ teaspoons tapioca flour*, mixed with
   1 tablespoon water (optional)
sea salt and freshly ground black pepper

* See Glossary

Place the shallot and thyme in a large saucepan
and pour in the wine. Bring to the boil over
medium–high heat and simmer until reduced by
two-thirds. Mix in the mustard, then pour in the
broth and return to the boil. Reduce the heat
to medium and simmer, occasionally skimming
the scum that rises to the surface, until the jus is
reduced by three-quarters and has a sauce-like
consistency. If the jus is still a little too thin, you
can thicken it slightly by whisking in the tapioca
mixture and simmering until it coats the back of
a spoon. Strain through a sieve and season with
salt and pepper. Store in an airtight container
in the fridge for up to 5 days or freeze for up to
3 months.

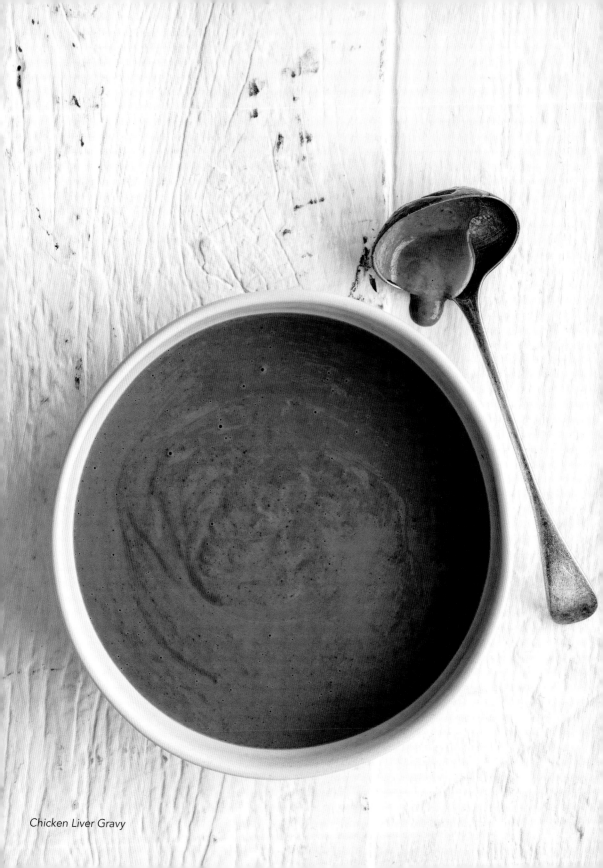

Chicken Liver Gravy

CHICKEN LIVER GRAVY

Makes 900 ml

500 g chicken livers (you can also use duck, lamb or calf's liver)
2 tablespoons coconut oil or good-quality animal fat*
1 onion, chopped
2 garlic cloves, finely chopped
3 portobello mushrooms, chopped
1 teaspoon finely chopped thyme leaves
1 litre Beef or Brown Chicken Bone Broth (page 165 or 166), plus extra if needed
sea salt and freshly ground black pepper

* See Glossary

Rinse the chicken livers under cold water and pat dry with paper towel. Trim off any fat, sinew and veins.

Melt the coconut oil or animal fat in a saucepan over medium heat. Add the onion and cook, stirring occasionally, for 8 minutes, or until softened and starting to caramelise. Stir in the garlic and cook for 1 minute, or until fragrant. Next, add the livers and cook for 3 minutes, or until browned but still pink on the inside. Remove the livers from the pan and set aside.

Add the mushroom and thyme to the pan, pour in the broth and bring to the boil. Reduce the heat to medium and simmer for 20 minutes, or until reduced by half.

Return the chicken livers to the pan and cook for 1 minute. Season with salt and pepper.

Blend the gravy with a hand-held or high-speed blender until smooth. Add more broth if you prefer a thinner gravy. Pass through a fine sieve and serve. Store in an airtight container in the fridge for up to 5 days or freeze for up to 3 months.

CHILLI OIL

Makes 300 ml

35 g chilli flakes
250 ml (1 cup) olive oil

Place the chilli flakes and olive oil in a small saucepan over low heat and gently stir for 5 minutes to warm through. Do not boil or the chilli will burn.

Allow to cool, then transfer to an airtight jar or bottle and store in the pantry for up to 3 months.

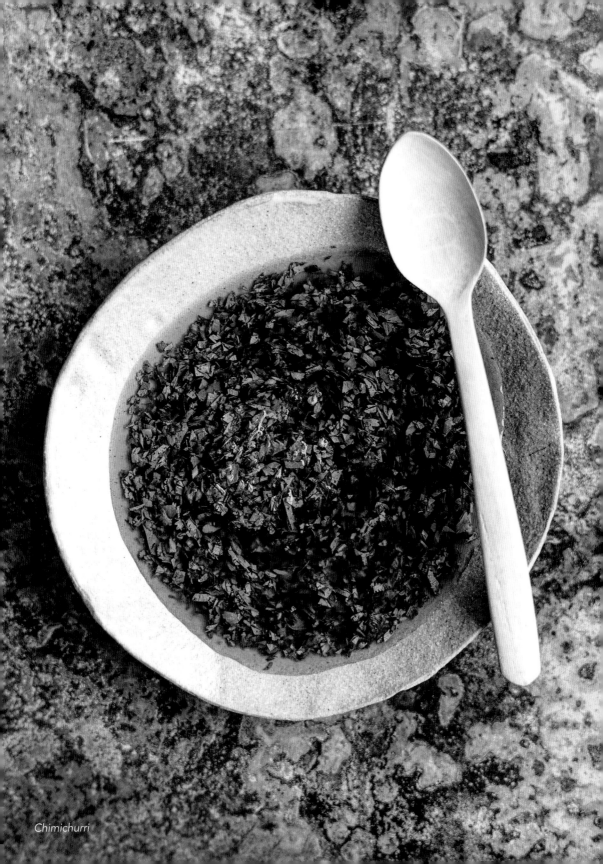

Chimichurri

CHIMICHURRI

Makes 450 ml

4 garlic cloves, peeled
sea salt
1 long red chilli, deseeded and finely chopped
  (leave the seeds in if you like it extra spicy)
2 very large handfuls of flat-leaf parsley leaves
2 very large handfuls of coriander leaves
80 ml (⅓ cup) apple cider vinegar
1 teaspoon ground cumin
250 ml (1 cup) extra-virgin olive oil
freshly ground black pepper

Place the garlic and a little salt in a mortar and
crush with the pestle. Add the chilli, parsley and
coriander and pound to a paste. Stir through
the vinegar, cumin and olive oil, then taste and
season with salt and pepper. Alternatively, place
the garlic, chilli and herbs in a food processor
and process until finely chopped. With the motor
running, pour in the vinegar and oil and process
to combine. Add the cumin and season with salt
and pepper. Store in an airtight container in the
fridge for up to 1 week.

COCONUT NAAN BREAD

Makes 6

100 g (1 cup) almond meal
125 g (1 cup) tapioca flour*
125 ml (½ cup) coconut milk
sea salt
coconut oil, for cooking

* See Glossary

Combine the almond meal, tapioca flour, coconut
milk and 125 ml (½ cup) of water in a bowl, mix
well and season with salt.

Heat a small non-stick frying pan over medium
heat. Add enough coconut oil to coat the surface
of the pan, then pour in 3 tablespoons of batter
and swirl around slightly. Cook for 2½ minutes, or
until mostly cooked through, then flip and cook
for 3 minutes, or until golden and crisp. Repeat
with the remaining mixture. Store in the fridge for
up to 1 week or freeze for up to 3 months.

CRISPY CURRY LEAVES

Makes 4 sprigs

150 ml melted coconut oil
4 fresh curry leaf sprigs
sea salt

Heat the coconut oil in a frying pan over medium
heat. Cooking in batches of two sprigs at a time,
add the curry leaves and fry for 4–5 seconds until
crisp. Remove with a slotted spoon and drain on
paper towel. Season with salt.

CRISPY SHALLOTS

Makes 2–4 tablespoons

250 ml (1 cup) melted coconut oil or
    good-quality animal fat*
4–8 French shallots, finely sliced

* See Glossary

Heat the coconut oil or animal fat in a small
saucepan over medium heat. Add the shallot
and cook for 2–3 minutes until golden. Remove
with a slotted spoon and drain on paper towel.
(You can re-use the oil for sautéing vegetables or
cooking meat, chicken or fish.) Store in an airtight
container in the pantry.

CURRY POWDER

Makes 130 g

3 tablespoons coriander seeds
2 tablespoons cumin seeds
2 tablespoons yellow mustard seeds
1 tablespoon fenugreek seeds
2 star anise
1 tablespoon allspice berries
3 heaped tablespoons ground turmeric

Combine the seeds, star anise and allspice
berries in a frying pan. Toast, tossing constantly,
over medium heat for 1–2 minutes until fragrant.
Remove from the heat and allow to cool.

Grind the toasted spices with the turmeric using
a spice grinder or mortar and pestle. Store in an
airtight container in the pantry for up to 3 months.

FERMENTED CHILLI SAMBAL

Makes 1 x 1 litre jar

800 g long red chillies
15 dried chillies
2 French shallots, chopped
5 garlic cloves, peeled
1 tablespoon finely grated ginger
½ teaspoon ground turmeric
1 tablespoon shrimp paste
2 teaspoons tamarind paste*
2 tablespoons coconut sugar
3 teaspoons sea salt
1 tablespoon fish sauce
125 ml (½ cup) filtered water

* See Glossary

You will need a 1.5 litre preserving jar with an
airlock lid for this recipe. Wash the jar and all the
utensils you will be using in very hot water or run
them through a hot rinse cycle in the dishwasher.

Place all the ingredients except the water in a
food processor and process until finely chopped.
Pour in the water and blend to a fine paste.
Spoon into the prepared jar, close the lid to seal,
then wrap a tea towel around the side of the jar
to block out the light; leave the airlock exposed.
Store in a dark place with a temperature of
16–23°C for 7–10 days. (You can place the jar in an
esky to maintain a more consistent temperature.)

After the chilli mixture has bubbled and brewed
for about a week, set a fine sieve over a bowl.
Tip in the chilli mixture and press down with
a wooden spoon to extract as much sauce as
possible (discard the leftover pulp). Pour into
a clean 1 litre jar and close the lid to seal.

The chilli sambal will keep in the fridge for
several months.

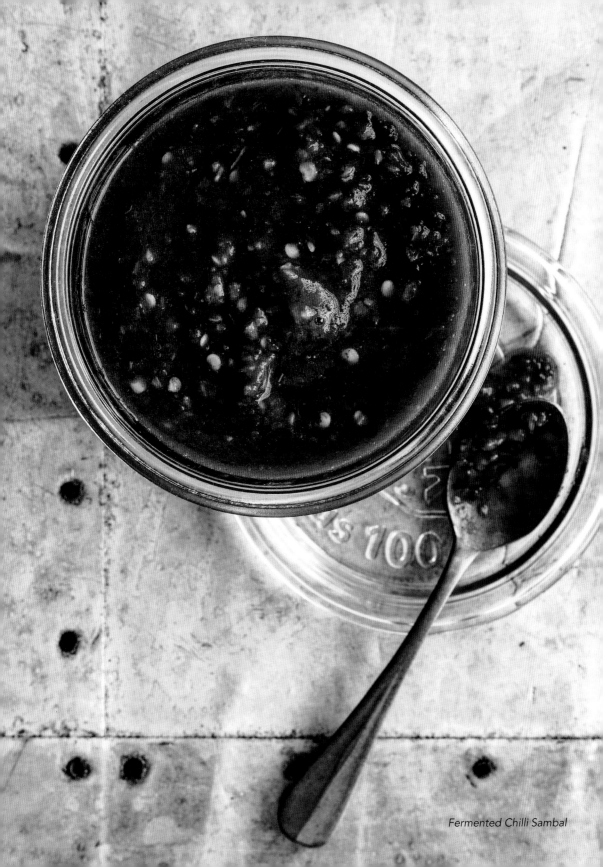

Fermented Chilli Sambal

FISH BONE BROTH

Makes 3 litres

3–4 non-oily fish carcasses and heads
   (such as snapper, barramundi or kingfish)
2 celery stalks, roughly chopped
2 onions, roughly chopped
1 carrot, roughly chopped
2 tablespoons apple cider vinegar
1 handful of thyme sprigs and flat-leaf
   parsley stalks
3 fresh bay leaves

Place the fish carcasses and heads in a stockpot, add the veggies and vinegar and cover with 3.5 litres of cold water. Bring to the boil, skimming off the scum that rises to the top. Tie the herbs together with kitchen string and add to the broth. Reduce the heat to low, cover and simmer for 3–4 hours.

Remove the fish carcasses and heads with tongs or a slotted spoon. Strain the broth through a fine sieve into storage containers. Cover and cool in the fridge. Remove the congealed fat that rises to the top (it is a fantastic, stable cooking fat) and store it in a glass container in the fridge for up to 2 weeks – use it for frying and sautéing. Transfer the gelatinous broth to smaller airtight containers and store for up to 4 days in the fridge or freeze for up to 3 months.

HOT SAUCE

Makes 500 ml

2 tablespoons coconut oil or good-quality
   animal fat*
1 onion, finely chopped
6 long red chillies, chopped
2–3 habanero chillies, deseeded and chopped
4 garlic cloves, finely chopped
3 tomatoes, chopped
200 ml apple cider vinegar
2 teaspoons sea salt
1 tablespoon honey
2 tablespoons tamari or coconut aminos*

* See Glossary

Heat the coconut oil or animal fat in a large saucepan over medium heat. Add the onion, chillies and garlic and cook for 5 minutes, or until softened. Reduce the heat to medium–low, then stir in the tomato, vinegar, salt, honey, tamari or coconut aminos and 3 tablespoons of water. Simmer, stirring occasionally, for about 30 minutes until the tomato breaks down and the flavour develops. Allow to cool.

Transfer the tomato and chilli mixture to a blender and blend until smooth. Strain through a fine sieve, if desired, discarding the leftover pulp. Pour the hot sauce into glass jars with screw-top lids and store in the fridge for up to 1 month.

HOISIN SAUCE

Makes about 220 ml

125 ml (½ cup) tamari or coconut aminos*
80 g raw honey
2 tablespoons tahini
¼ teaspoon chinese five spice
sea salt and freshly ground black pepper

* See Glossary

Place all the ingredients in a bowl and mix until smooth. Store in an airtight glass jar in the fridge for up to 3 weeks.

PICKLED RED ONION

Makes 300 g

1 red onion, cut into 12 wedges
125 ml (½ cup) red wine vinegar
2 fresh bay leaves
1 tablespoon honey
sea salt and freshly ground black pepper

Place the onion, vinegar, bay leaves and honey in a small saucepan and bring to a simmer over medium heat. Cover with a lid and cook for 1 minute, then remove from the heat and allow to cool completely. Season with salt and pepper. Store in an airtight glass container in the fridge for up to 2 months.

PIZZA SAUCE

Makes 400 ml

400 g whole peeled tomatoes (see Note
   page 66)
1 teaspoon dried oregano
2 pinches of freshly ground black pepper
sea salt

Combine all the ingredients in a food processor
and process until smooth. Season with salt to
taste. Store in an airtight container in the fridge
for up to 4 days.

RED WINE JUS

Makes 600 ml

2 tablespoons coconut oil or good-quality
   animal fat*, melted
100 g French shallots, sliced
2 garlic cloves, lightly crushed
6 thyme sprigs
3 tablespoons tomato paste
600 ml dry red wine (such as shiraz)
3 litres Beef Bone Broth (page 165)
sea salt and freshly ground black pepper

* See Glossary

Melt 1 tablespoon of the coconut oil or animal
fat in a saucepan over medium–high heat. Add
the shallot and sauté, stirring occasionally, for
5 minutes, or until lightly caramelised. Add the
garlic, thyme and tomato paste and continue to
cook for 1 minute. Pour in the wine, bring to the
boil and simmer until reduced by two-thirds.

Add the broth to the pan and return to the boil.
Turn down the heat to medium and simmer,
occasionally skimming the scum that rises to
the surface, until the jus is reduced by about
85 per cent (to leave 600 ml) and has a sauce-like
consistency. Strain through a sieve and season
with salt and pepper. Store in an airtight container
in the fridge for up to 3 weeks or freeze for up to
3 months.

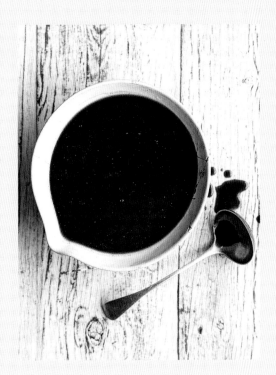

Red Wine Jus

QUICK PICKLED GARLIC

Makes 8 cloves

8 garlic cloves, roughly chopped
125 ml (½ cup) apple cider vinegar
½ teaspoon sea salt

Place all the ingredients in a small saucepan, add 2 tablespoons of water and bring to a simmer over medium heat. Reduce the heat to low, cover with the lid and gently simmer for 15 minutes, or until semi-tender. Remove from the heat and allow to cool completely. Strain, reserving the pickling liquid if needed.

RENDERED ANIMAL FAT

Makes up to 600 g

1 kg pork back fat, beef fat, lamb fat, duck skin or chicken skin (see Note)
125 ml (½ cup) filtered water

If using pork, beef or lamb fat, trim any flesh from the fat and cut the fat into 2 cm dice.

Place the fat or skin and filtered water in a large saucepan over low heat and simmer, stirring occasionally (taking care as the fat may spit), for 3½–4 hours until the water has evaporated and the fat is golden brown and liquefied. Try and keep the fat at around 100°C (use a candy thermometer to test the temperature). You will notice little solid bits of brown crackling floating to the surface and a lot of clear liquid; this is an indication that the fat has rendered and is ready to be taken off the heat.

Allow the rendered fat to cool a little before straining through a fine sieve into containers or ice-cube trays. Save the leftover crackling bits as they make a delicious snack. The cooled melted fat will be creamy white in colour. Store in an airtight container in the fridge for up to 1 month or freeze for up to 6 months.

NOTE

You can buy animal fat or skin from your butcher. They may need to be ordered in advance.

SMOKED LARD

Makes 500 g–1 kg

500 g–1 kg lard (see Rendered Animal Fat, below left)
1 kg hickory or apple wood chips, soaked in water for 1–2 hours, drained

Place the lard in a roasting tin.

Divide the soaked wood chips between two aluminium barbecue trays. Place one tray under the barbecue grill grates, directly on the heat source, in a far corner. Set the other tray aside.

Turn all the barbecue burners to high, cover with the lid and preheat to 180–200°C. At this stage the wood chips will begin to smoke. Turn off the middle burners and allow the temperature to drop to 100°C. Quickly place the lard on the middle grate, away from the heat, then close the lid. Reduce the other burners to low and maintain the heat at no higher than 100°C. Smoke the lard for 3 hours, switching the barbecue trays when the smoke starts to die down (halfway through the process). You may notice that the wood chips turn to ash – this is the signal to change trays. Remove the melted smoked lard from the barbecue and pour into a heatproof bowl. Cool and store in an airtight glass jar in the fridge for up to 1 month or freeze for up to 6 months.

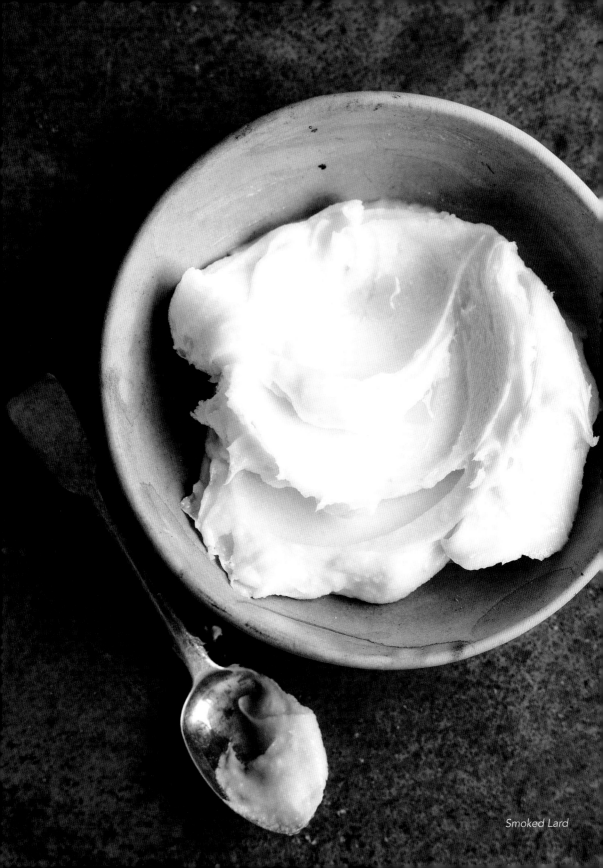

Smoked Lard

SMOKY BARBECUE SAUCE

Makes 420 g

100 g tomato paste
3 tablespoons apple cider vinegar
1 tablespoon Dijon mustard
120 g honey
100 ml maple syrup
½ teaspoon smoked paprika
100 ml tamari or coconut aminos*
2 garlic cloves, finely chopped
1½ tablespoons liquid smoke (see Note)
    (optional)
1 pinch of ground cloves
1 cinnamon stick
sea salt (optional)

* See Glossary

Place all the ingredients in a saucepan over medium heat, mix well and bring to a simmer. Reduce the heat to low and cook, stirring occasionally, for 10 minutes. Season with salt, if desired, and allow to cool. Remove the cinnamon stick and store the sauce in an airtight container in the fridge for up to 2 weeks.

NOTE

Liquid smoke is a water-soluble liquid that forms from condensed smoke particles when chips from a hardwood (such as hickory) are burned. You can buy it from some supermarkets, delis, specialty food stores or online.

TEXAS-STYLE BARBECUE SAUCE

Makes 600 ml

125 ml (½ cup) melted Smoked Lard (page 176)
1 onion, chopped
1 celery stalk, finely chopped
3 garlic cloves, finely chopped
125 ml (½ cup) apple cider vinegar
250 ml (1 cup) Tomato Ketchup (page 179)
120 ml filtered water
3 tablespoons Worcestershire sauce
1 teaspoon tapioca flour*, mixed with
    1 tablespoon water
½ teaspoon freshly ground black pepper
1 teaspoon chilli powder

Place the smoked lard in a saucepan over medium heat. Add the onion and celery and sauté for 5 minutes, or until softened. Stir in the garlic and cook for 1 minute, or until fragrant.

Add the vinegar, tomato ketchup, filtered water, Worcestershire sauce, tapioca mixture, pepper and chilli powder to the pan and bring to the boil. Turn down the heat and simmer for 15 minutes, or until reduced and thickened. Remove from the heat and allow to cool.

Transfer the sauce to a blender and blend until smooth. Pass through a fine strainer and season with more salt and pepper if needed. Store in an airtight container in the fridge for up to 3 weeks.

TIP

This sauce is best served at room temperature, as the lard causes it to solidify when refrigerated. Gently warm the sauce on the stovetop and whisk until smooth before using.

TOMATO KETCHUP

Makes 330 g

180 g tomato paste
100 ml filtered water
2 tablespoons apple cider vinegar
1 teaspoon garlic powder
1 teaspoon onion powder
½ teaspoon ground cinnamon
¼ teaspoon freshly grated nutmeg
2 teaspoons honey
pinch of ground cloves

Mix the tomato paste and water in a small saucepan. Place over medium heat and bring to a simmer (add more water if you prefer your sauce to be thinner). Remove from the heat and stir in the remaining ingredients until incorporated and smooth. Cool and store in an airtight glass jar in the fridge for up to 4 weeks.

TYPHOON GARLIC

Makes 90 g

150 g garlic cloves (about 50), peeled
400 ml melted coconut oil
sea salt

Place the garlic in the bowl of a food processor and process until finely chopped. Don't over-process as it will turn to mush.

Combine the garlic and coconut oil in a saucepan over medium heat and cook, stirring constantly, for 5–10 minutes, or until the garlic is lightly golden and crispy. (The garlic can burn very quickly so remove the pan from the heat as soon as it turns pale golden.) Strain the garlic (reserve the oil for use in other recipes), shaking off any excess oil. Drain on paper towel and season with salt.

The garlic can be stored in an airtight container in the pantry for up to 1 month. The oil can be stored in a jar in the fridge for up to 1 month and can be used for any kind of cooking.

VIETNAMESE PICKLED CARROT, CUCUMBER AND DAIKON

Makes 1 x 1 litre jar

180 ml apple cider vinegar
150 ml filtered water
2 tablespoons honey
1¼ teaspoons sea salt
2 tablespoons fish sauce
2 carrots (about 200 g), cut into matchsticks
¼ daikon (about 125 g), cut into matchsticks
3 Lebanese cucumbers, halved lengthways, deseeded and cut into matchsticks
3 garlic cloves, finely chopped
½ teaspoon finely grated ginger
1½ tablespoons finely chopped coriander roots and stalks
2 long red chillies, 1 cut into matchsticks and 1 finely chopped

You will need a 1 litre glass jar with an airtight lid for this recipe. Wash the jar and all the utensils you will be using in very hot water or run them through a hot rinse cycle in the dishwasher.

Combine the vinegar, filtered water, honey, salt and fish sauce in a large bowl and mix well.

In another bowl, combine the carrot, daikon, cucumber, garlic, ginger, coriander and chilli, then gently mix.

Fill the prepared jar with the vegetable mixture, then pour in the pickling liquid. The vegetables should be completely submerged in the liquid. Cover with the lid and place in the fridge for at least 1 day. For best results, and to allow the veggies to become more flavourful and tangy, pickle for 3–4 days. Once opened, the pickled veggies submerged in the liquid will keep in the fridge for up to 3 weeks.

GLOSSARY

Coconut aminos

Made from coconut sap, coconut aminos is similar in flavour to a light soy sauce. Because it is free of both soy and gluten, it makes a great alternative to soy sauce and tamari. Coconut aminos is available at health-food stores.

Coconut oil

Coconut oil is extracted from the meat of mature coconuts. It has a high smoke point, making it great for cooking at high temperatures. The viscosity of coconut oil changes depending on the temperature and ranges from liquid to solid. Although coconut oil is high in saturated fats, they are mainly medium-chain saturated fatty acids, which means the body can use them quickly and does not have to store them. Coconut oil is available from supermarkets and health-food stores. Look for virgin cold-pressed varieties, as these have had the least amount of processing.

Gelatine

Gelatine is the cooked form of collagen, which is a protein found in bones, skin and connective tissue. I always choose gelatine sourced from organic, grass-fed beef, such as Great Lakes Gelatin Company. Vegetarian substitutes for gelatine include agar agar and carrageen, which are made from two different types of seaweed. Sometimes these aren't as strong as regular gelatine, so you may need to increase the quantity. Some kosher gelatines are also vegan. You can buy gelatine made from organic, grass-fed beef, agar agar and carrageen from health-food stores or online.

Good-quality animal fat

I use either coconut oil or good-quality animal fats for cooking as they have high smoke points (meaning they do not oxidise at high temperatures). Some of my favourite animal fats to use are lard (pork fat), tallow (rendered beef fat), rendered chicken fat and duck fat. These may be hard to find – ask at your local butcher or meat supplier, look online for meat suppliers who sell them or make your own (see page 176).

Jarred fish

I buy preserved fish – such as anchovies, tuna, salmon, mackerel and sardines – in jars rather than cans, due to the presence of Bisphenol A (BPA) in many cans. BPA is a toxic chemical that can interfere with our hormonal system. You can find jarred fish at specialty food stores and supermarkets.

Makrut lime leaves

More commonly known as kaffir lime leaves, the term makrut lime is becoming more widely used these days as the word 'kaffir' is offensive in many cultures.

Nori

Nori is a dark green, paper-like, toasted seaweed used for most kinds of sushi and other Japanese dishes. Nori provides an abundance of essential nutrients and is rich in vitamins, iron, minerals, amino acids, omega-3 and omega-6, and antioxidants. Nori sheets are commonly used to roll sushi, but they can also be added to salads, soups, and fish, meat and vegetable dishes. You can buy nori sheets from Asian grocers and most supermarkets.

Nutritional yeast

Nutritional yeast is a source of complete protein and vitamins, in particular B-complex vitamins. It contains thiamine, folates, niacin, selenium, zinc and riboflavin, making it a highly nutritious addition to your diet.

Pomegranate molasses

Pomegranate molasses is a thick, tangy and glossy reduction of pomegranate juice that is rich in antioxidants. Pomegranate molasses is used in Middle Eastern countries for glazing meat and chicken before roasting, and in sauces, salad dressings and marinades. You can buy it from Middle Eastern grocers and some delis.

Psyllium husks

Psyllium, also known as ispaghula, is a gluten-free, soluble fibre produced from the *Plantago ovata* plant, native to India and Pakistan. Psyllium is an indigestible dietary fibre and is primarily used to maintain intestinal health, as the high fibre content absorbs excess liquid in the gut. When exposed to liquids, the husks swell up to create a gel. It is therefore important to drink plenty of fluids when consuming psyllium. Psyllium products can be found at health-food stores and some supermarkets.

Salt

I use sea salt or Himalayan salt in my cooking, as they are less processed than table salt, contain more minerals and have a lovely crunchy texture. Himalayan salt is light pink in colour due to the presence of a number of different minerals, including iron, magnesium, calcium and copper. You can buy sea salt and Himalayan salt at supermarkets and health-food stores.

Sweeteners

Erythritol

Erythritol is a naturally derived sugar substitute, produced by a fermentation process, that looks and tastes very much like sugar, yet has almost no calories. It comes in granulated and powdered forms. Erythritol has been used in Japan since 1990 in sweets, chocolate, yoghurt, fillings, jellies, jams, beverages, and as a sugar substitute. Erythritol is classified as a sugar alcohol. Sugar alcohols, also called polyols, are sugar substitutes that are either extracted from plants or manufactured from starches. Buy online and from health-food stores.

Monk fruit sweetener

Monk fruit is a small, green gourd that resembles a melon. It is grown in South-East Asia. The fruit was first used by Buddhist monks in the 13th century, hence the fruit's unusual name. Monk fruit sweeteners are made from the fruit's extract. They may be blended with dextrose or other ingredients to balance sweetness. Monk fruit extract is 150–200 times sweeter than sugar. The extract contains zero calories and zero carbohydrates. Monk fruit sweetener can be found online and in health-food stores.

Stevia

Native to South America, stevia grows into a shrub with naturally sweet leaves. The sweet extraction has no calories and is over 100 times sweeter than cane sugar. Stevia leaves have been used by the people of Brazil and Paraguay for hundreds of years as a means of sweetening food. Stevia is also believed to provide relief from skin irritations. You can find stevia in most supermarkets.

Xylitol

Xylitol is a sugar alcohol found in fruits and vegetables. It is low in carbohydrates and slowly absorbed, so has a minimal effect on blood sugar, making it useful for people wishing to avoid sugar. You can find granulated xylitol in health-food stores and some supermarkets.

Tamarind paste

Tamarind paste is made from the pods of the tamarind tree and is used as a souring agent, particularly in Indian dishes, chutneys and curries. It is also used as an ingredient in sauces and side dishes for pork, chicken and fish. It can be found at Asian grocers and some supermarkets.

Tapioca flour

Tapioca flour is made by grinding up the dried root of the manioc (also known as cassava) plant. It can be used to thicken dishes or in gluten-free baking. In Australia, arrowroot and tapioca flour are considered the same, even though they are actually from different plants. You can find tapioca flour and arrowroot at health-food stores and some supermarkets.

Vegetable starter culture

Vegetable starter culture is a preparation used to kickstart the fermentation process when culturing vegetables and yoghurts. I use a broad-spectrum starter sourced from organic vegetables rather than one grown from dairy sources, as this ensures the highest number of living, active bacteria and produces consistently successful results free of pathogens. Vegetable starter culture usually comes in sachets and can be purchased from health-food stores or online. You can also get fresh, non-dairy starter cultures for yoghurt and kefir (we recommend kulturedwellness.com).

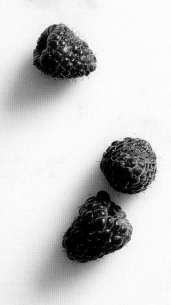

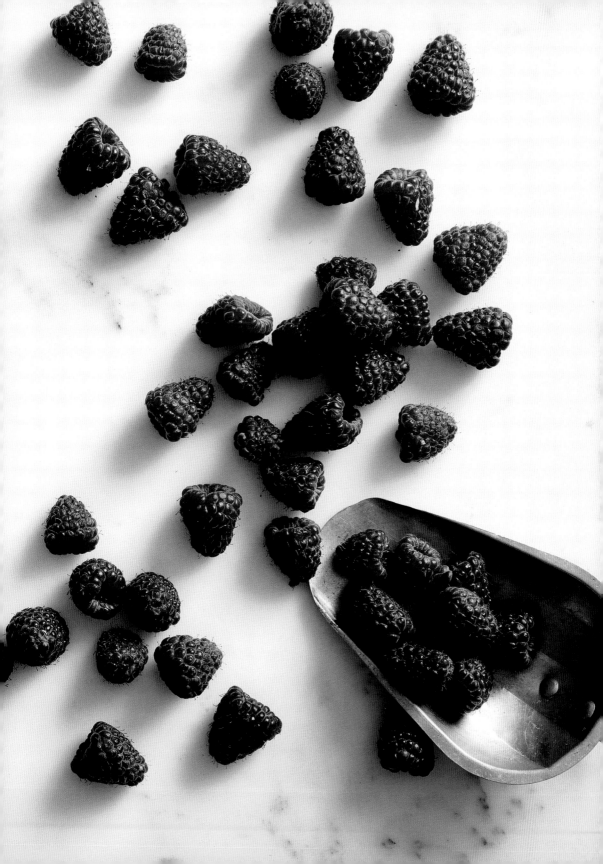

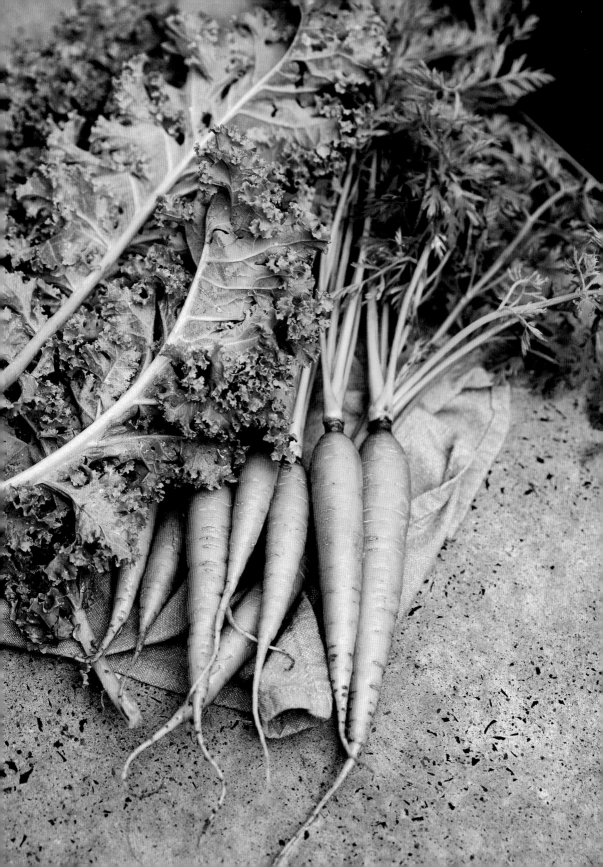

CONVERSION CHARTS

Measuring cups and spoons may vary slightly from one country to another, but the difference is generally not enough to affect a recipe. All cup and spoon measures are level.

One Australian metric measuring cup holds 250 ml (8 fl oz), one Australian metric tablespoon holds 20 ml (4 teaspoons) and one Australian metric teaspoon holds 5 ml. North America, New Zealand and the UK use a 15 ml (3-teaspoon) tablespoon.

LENGTH

METRIC	IMPERIAL
3 mm	⅛ inch
6 mm	¼ inch
1 cm	½ inch
2.5 cm	1 inch
5 cm	2 inches
18 cm	7 inches
20 cm	8 inches
23 cm	9 inches
25 cm	10 inches
30 cm	12 inches

LIQUID MEASURES

ONE AMERICAN PINT	ONE IMPERIAL PINT
500 ml (16 fl oz)	600 ml (20 fl oz)

CUP	METRIC	IMPERIAL
⅛ cup	30 ml	1 fl oz
¼ cup	60 ml	2 fl oz
⅓ cup	80 ml	2½ fl oz
½ cup	125 ml	4 fl oz
⅔ cup	160 ml	5 fl oz
¾ cup	180 ml	6 fl oz
1 cup	250 ml	8 fl oz
2 cups	500 ml	16 fl oz
2¼ cups	560 ml	20 fl oz
4 cups	1 litre	32 fl oz

DRY MEASURES

The most accurate way to measure dry ingredients is to weigh them. However, if using a cup, add the ingredient loosely to the cup and level with a knife; don't compact the ingredient unless the recipe requests 'firmly packed'.

METRIC	IMPERIAL
15 g	½ oz
30 g	1 oz
60 g	2 oz
125 g	4 oz (¼ lb)
185 g	6 oz
250 g	8 oz (½ lb)
375 g	12 oz (¾ lb)
500 g	16 oz (1 lb)
1 kg	32 oz (2 lb)

OVEN TEMPERATURES

CELSIUS	FAHRENHEIT	CELSIUS	GAS MARK
100°C	200°F	110°C	¼
120°C	250°F	130°C	½
150°C	300°F	140°C	1
160°C	325°F	150°C	2
180°C	350°F	170°C	3
200°C	400°F	180°C	4
220°C	425°F	190°C	5
		200°C	6
		220°C	7
		230°C	8
		240°C	9
		250°C	10

THANKS

A mountain of gratitude to my glorious family, especially my wonderful wife, Nic, and my two amazing daughters, Indii and Chilli. You three angels are a constant source of pure inspiration and happiness, and it is a humbling honour to walk beside you all throughout this life. Thank you for being your bright, fun-loving, authentic and unconditionally loving selves.

To the absolute wonder twins, Monica and Jacinta Cannataci, you both add your own magic essence to everything we create together, and this book just wouldn't be the same without your input. Thank you both for working so graciously and tirelessly, and for all that you do!

To the incredible photography and styling team of William Meppem, Rob Palmer, Steve Brown and Lucy Tweed. You all bring a unique sense of beauty that never ceases to be exceptionally pleasing, and I'm endlessly thankful to you all.

To Kylie Bailey, thank you so much for helping get this book to where it is now. So many people will benefit greatly from all your hard work.

To Ingrid Ohlsson and Mary Small, thank you for passionately orchestrating the path that allows so much goodness to come to life. It is a pleasure to work with you both, always!

Thanks to Clare Marshall, for making sure everything is as it should be. It is a joy to have you across all the details.

To Clare Keighery, thanks for being the best publicist any author could wish to work with.

To Megan Johnston, thank you for your careful and thorough editing.

To Kirby Armstrong, thank you for creating such a gorgeous design for the book.

A very warm thank you to my sweet mum, Joy. Among many things, you passed on your love of cooking and there's no doubt that I wouldn't be where I am without you.

I also wish to express a huge thank you to my teachers, peers, mentors and friends, who are all genuinely working towards creating a healthier world and who are all in their own right true forces for good: Nora Gedgaudas and Lisa Collins, Trevor Hendy, Rudy Eckhardt, Dr Pete Bablis, Dr David Perlmutter, Dr Alessio Fasano, Dr Kelly Brogan, Dr William Davis, Dr Joseph Mercola, Helen Padarin, Dr Natasha Campbell-McBride, Dr Frank Lipman, Dr Libby, Prof. Tim Noakes, Pete Melov and Prof. Martha Herbert, to name a few.